Beyond the Shadows

Beyond the Shadows

EILEEN MITSON

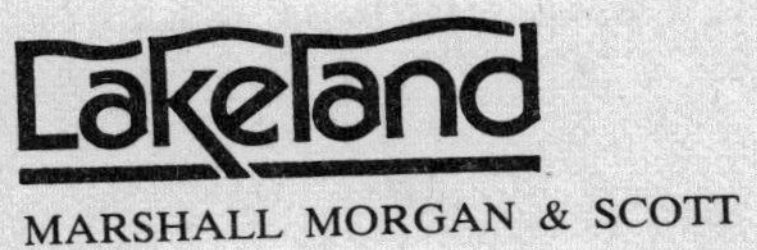

MARSHALL MORGAN & SCOTT

Lakeland
Marshall Morgan & Scott
1 Bath Street, London EC1V 9LB

First published 1968
First paperback edition 1973
Reprinted
Impression number 10 9 8 7 6 5 4

ISBN 0 551 00469 X

Printed in Great Britain by
J. W. Arrowsmith Ltd., Bristol

DEDICATED

to the memory of

FRANKIE

the heroine of this story

Not dead – oh, no, but borne beyond the shadows
Into the full, clear light;
Forever done with mist and cloud and tempest
Where all is calm and bright.

Not even sleeping – called to glad awakening
In Heaven's cloudless day:
Not still and moveless – stepped from earth's rough places
To walk the King's highway.

Not silent – just passed out of earthly hearing
To sing Heaven's sweet new song;
Not lonely – dearly loved and dearly loving
Amid the white-robed throng.

But not forgetful – keeping fond remembrance
Of dear one's left awhile;
And looking gladly to the bright re-union
With hand-clasp and with smile.

Oh, no, not dead, but past all fear of dying,
And with all suffering o'er;
Say not that I am dead when Jesus calls me
To live for evermore.

Chapter 1

On an evening in late July, green with slanting rain, I sat by the window and read an article about a little girl who had died of leukaemia.

As I read, the awful pathos of this story seeped into my spirit. What could be more bitter than this? To know for a year, or even more, that your child must die; to nurse her through a sickness for which there is no known cure; to keep this knowledge locked away in your broken heart, lest the child guess at your grief; to watch her pass slowly from the bright plains of childhood into the valley of the shadow of death . . . How could any mother bear such torture?

Turning over these thoughts in my mind that summer's evening, I allowed my imagination full play. Living the part of the mother in the article, I suddenly asked myself a question. What if this should happen to me? What if one of my children, at that moment sleeping safely in their beds, should fall prey to such a monster of disease? The chance must be one in several thousand, and this was the kind of thing which happened only to the unfortunate stranger – never to oneself. . . .

But what if it should? Would I accept such a blow as being 'the perfect will of God?' Would my faith stand the test? Would I, in my over-sensitivity, my inherent cowardice, be given a supernatural strength to live through such an experience? Would the fact that I was a believing Christian really make so much difference?

And then a new idea was born. What if I wrote a novel around this theme? What if I told the story of an imaginary family who, in Christ's strength, faced and triumphed over such a tragedy as this. . . . The idea filled me with excitement. I decided to keep the article so as to have the facts of a real leukaemia case ready at hand. When I had finished writing the novel I was working upon at the time, then I would think again about this new story. In the meantime, it could go into cold storage.

That was two years ago. Today, as I begin this story, I remember that article, so full of useful facts, and I remember how my imagination was so ready to project itself into that other mother's experience. But I no longer need the facts, nor do I need to play any tricks with my imagination.

For the story that I now write is autobiography, not a novel; it is fact, not fiction, and I am the mother in the story.

But let us begin at the beginning, on a Sunday afternoon in November, 1954 . . .

'It's a girl,' said the midwife absently, her mind on other things.

'It can't be,' I protested weakly, surfacing gratefully for the last time from the analgesia. 'The only name we've thought of is Christopher John.'

'Then you'll have to think again, quick, Mum, 'cause Christopher's not going to do for this one! Is it, my little love?' – as a thin wail zigzagged into the quiet room. 'Here, take her for a minute, there's a good girl.'

As I looked down into the crumpled features, a strange new sensation seemed to spread itself through my whole being. I tried to name it, to think backwards over the two and a half years to the time when Elizabeth had been born, but the feeling was like nothing I had ever experienced before. It was nothing as simple as relief, relaxation, or a sense of achievement; nor was it merely maternal joy. The more I tried to take hold of the emotion and to analyse it, the more elusive it became.

'She's just like you,' I told Arthur, as he bent over the child in my arms. 'Look at her lovely wide brow, and her little short nose!'

As I sipped the cup of tea he had brought me, I thought, 'Maybe that's it. Maybe it's because she looks so much like her Daddy that I felt as I did . . .' I remembered how I had longed that our first child would be like Arthur, and how disappointed I had been at first when I saw that her nose was a replica of mine! But the little one in my arms was a Mitson to the very last detail.

'What are we going to call her?' I said now.

'We'll think of something,' Arthur said cheerfully. 'The only thing that matters at the moment is that she's safely here!'

Suddenly, I was hungry. But later, I only pecked at the tastefully prepared meal he brought me. All at once, I wanted to be alone with my new baby, and with the strange emotion which still seemed to hover somewhere just over my head.

'Do you mind?' I said apologetically, handing Arthur the half-eaten meal. 'I think I could just do with a little sleep.'

Alone in the room, I savoured the moment to the full. There is a loneliness in birth, I thought, that even one's dearest cannot quite enter. Modern husbands may sit and hold one's hand throughout, may share the thrill of the moment of birth, and yet there is a point beyond which only the mother may pass. It is as though, no matter how fleetingly, she enters into a place which has the dimensions of eternity. Caught up inescapably into the miracle of new life, even the commonest of us are transformed by the experience, and in the moment of transformation, we are alone.

The transformation does not last. But the puzzling 'awareness' – (for want of a better word) – which hung about me as I gazed again into the face of my second daughter, did last, on and off, throughout the ten short years of her life. It was like a phrase of music being played at the most unexpected moments, almost out of earshot, but not quite . . .

When, shortly before she died, I held her once more in my arms, as I had held her, then, on that grey Sunday afternoon in November, when she was but a few minutes old, I tasted again the quiet, inexplicable exaltation, and I believe I understood at last.

Chapter 2

In case anyone should be led to think, on reading the rest of this story, that Arthur and I were anything more or less than ordinary, flesh-and-blood parents – that we were somehow thicker-skinned or less sensitive than average, a brief sketch of our background may serve to show that, if anything, the opposite is true.

Arthur and I were born within eight miles of one another, but we searched pretty thoroughly for each other, without knowing it, for a number of years, and in a variety of places before we finally met.

I understand that the world dislikes a misfit, but I suppose that we both answered to that description at the time when our paths eventually crossed. And since most misfits stay that way for the rest of their lives, I can only suggest that a square peg ceases to be a problem either to itself, or to others when once it succeeds in finding itself a square hole! This, roughly, has been the situation with us.

Arthur and I had both been brought up in the evangelical faith, and in our teens had both experienced the 'new birth' which we believe the Bible teaches to be a necessity for salvation and eternal life. At the same time, we both became gradually aware of a kind of crippling sensitivity in ourselves, an artistic response to life which seemed to isolate us from those around us.

We discovered that most evangelicals had very little interest in the arts, and that some of the older ones even regarded such things as poetry and painting (unless used as a medium of expression for religious experience) as distinctly suspect. Fortunately, today there is a movement away from this attitude.

In those days, however, these things baffled and worried us – as young Christians, each in our separate corners, for we had not yet met. Arthur was reaching out towards a more abstract form of expression in art, and several of his paintings were hung in London galleries. I was writing poetry and allegories, and, after a spell of secretarial work in London, was struggling to read for a degree at home, with the vague hope of one day becoming a writer. We were both beginning to despair of ever finding someone with whom we could share our own peculiar religious and aesthetic experience.

So that when our mutual friends, Ray and Coral Guthrie, introduced us to each other at a 'Squash' for young people I had arranged at my parents' home in Essex, we were immediately drawn to one another. We could hardly believe, later, that Ray and Coral had had no thought of 'match-making' when they brought us together, so unlikely was it, humanly speaking, that we should ever have met otherwise!

Looking back, now, at the letters we wrote one another before our marriage – some rather highbrow ones at first, before the actual love letters began! – I think of the years between, and of how our love has grown into a strong tree, nurtured by the sunlight of mutual joys, and watered by the tears of shared sorrow. Viewing those early years in the light of future events, one is amazed by the slowly unfolding pattern in which nothing – not even the smallest event – seems to have happened by chance, or to have no part in the existing whole.

When we had been married for seven years, and our daughters were aged six and four, Arthur entered the London Bible College to train for the ministry. The call had come some two or three years earlier, but having studied at home for his University Entrance, Arthur had been prevented from going ahead with his plans by various family responsibilities and complications with his business.

But the day finally came when we moved into two rooms in a London suburb, kindly rented to us by a friend's mother at a very low figure. As friends were constantly reminding us, it was 'a big step to take', especially as it had meant abandoning a business carefully built up over the years, and selling up our home.

To move with two small children from a seven-roomed house of one's own into two partly furnished rooms, was in itself no small thing. But God provided wonderfully for all our various needs, and in spite of the restrictions involved, the next two years were happy ones. Elizabeth and Frances (or Frankie, as she was usually called) quickly adapted themselves to the new way of life, Arthur did well at his exams, and in August 1960 he was invited to the Pastorate of the Sewell Memorial Free Church in the lovely village of Lindfield, in Sussex.

Once more, it was through our friends Ray and Coral that we were introduced to this work. They had moved to Sussex some years before, and we were happy to know that our new home would be only a few miles from theirs.

It had been a long journey, but infinitely worthwhile. We had learned many valuable lessons, and above all, had proved the blessed reward of obeying the injunction given to us as a text at our wedding service:

'Whatsoever He saith unto you, *do it.*'

One day, when we had been in Lindfield for about two years, we received a telephone call from the eldest son of Ray and Coral. Ray had been taken into hospital with a thrombosis. He was forty-six at this time, and a full-time worker for the Caravan Mission to Village Children. He and Arthur were still close friends – their common interest in art had always bound them together. The day after this shattering phone call, we received another. I took this message, and to my horror heard David say: 'Father has gone.'

I cannot describe what this meant to us both at the time. For days I asked myself *'Why?'* I tried to imagine what I would have done if it had been Arthur – who was, after all, only about five years younger, and had very much the same kind of temperament.

When I went to see Coral, I was amazed to find her almost radiant. She talked with calm serenity of all that had happened, and of the joy that her loved one was now experiencing in the presence of God. Only once, just as I was leaving, did she break down and weep. Her witness to God's upholding power shook me profoundly. I could see that this was a *positive* thing; not just a 'bearing-up', but a visible, God-given peace of mind and heart.

Dimly I was aware that I had a whole lot of thinking to do. How often, speaking at women's meetings up and down the county, had I spoken of the power of the risen Christ to transform our daily experience, to carry us through trouble, to sustain us in grief. But now that I had seen this power in action, I was staggered beyond all thought. *How could she be like that?* This was the burning question. Yes, I knew that Christ was upholding her, but how could this really alter the suffering through which she must be passing? How could this consciousness of Christ's presence fill the empty chair? How could it help her to face the daily reminders that her beloved had gone?

Finally, I decided quite simply that she was made of different stuff from me. From this I drew comfort, for I told myself that God would never ask me to go through an experience like this – He knew I was not emotionally equipped for it. 'He will not suffer thee to be tempted (or tried) above that ye are able.' I rested in that.

But some time after this, the same challenge came to me in a different way. There had been – as there always seems to be nowadays – some trouble abroad. The papers were full of accounts of brutalities and violent death. As always, the innocent had suffered with the guilty; horror and grief and suffering now engulfed yet another section of struggling humanity.

Again, I asked myself: 'What if any of these things should happen to me?' My whole being recoiled in fear. I thought of missionaries who suffered and died at the hands of tormentors in the lands they had sacrificed all to evangelize. Could anything take away the terror from the heart of a man or woman who knew that at any moment death – and brutal death at that – would strike? How could being a Christian make any real difference? How could it?

After all, pain was pain. If you hit your head on the wall hard enough, it hurt – nothing could alter that. And if your husband or child died, then grief would strike you down. Grief was a normal, human reaction to the loss of a loved one. How could being a Christian make any difference, fundamentally, to that? I had seen Coral showing an amazing courage, seemingly triumphing over her grief, but how did I know that this was not somehow the numbing effect of great shock? Surely, inevitably, there would be a reaction? After all, Coral was only human.

But as the weeks and the months went by, Coral was still witnessing to others concerning the wonder of God's sustaining power and strength. Oh, yes, she had days when the way was hard, I knew that. But quite obviously the triumph I had seen was real.

And frankly, I could not understand it.

Chapter 3

It will be seen that the challenge 'How would *I* make out?' was becoming a recurring question in my mind, for it was not long after the events just described that I read the article about leukaemia. Perhaps my resolve to write a story about a family who had this tragedy to face was, in fact, my personal way of working this thing out for myself. Perhaps I thought that out of my own creative resources the answer would come. I do not know.

But it was almost immediately after this that Frankie began to complain of occasional aching legs. As a child, I had often suffered from 'leg-ache', and remembered my mother rubbing the backs of my knees with warm olive oil. So I did not worry unduly when Frankie woke up in the night and complained that her leg hurt.

Then one day she burst in from school with terror on her face, threw herself into my arms and said: 'Mummy, why do I feel so sad?'

With an effort I tried to jolly her out of it. She quietened down, ate a little dinner, and went back to school. But I could not forget the look of terror on her face – the face which was usually crinkled and dimpled with smiles. Frankie's smile was almost a byword in the village. It was a smile which lit up her round face and made her blue eyes shine, and dimples appear in her cheeks. It was amazing how many fathers of her school friends, as well as the mothers, fell unashamedly in love with her. 'There's just something about her,' I was told on more than one occasion – 'an imp and an angel rolled into one!'

So that the bouts of depression which now began to trouble her were terrifyingly abnormal. In May of 1964, Frankie began to complain more and more with her legs. Mostly, the trouble seemed centred in the left leg, but occasionally the other leg would be affected too. Although she never really made much fuss about this – usually telling me with a grin that her leg was hurting a bit – when she also began to say that her left eye hurt badly, I again approached the doctor. Up till now his diagnosis had been 'growing pains', but now he arranged for her to have her eyes tested, and also to have an X-ray on her leg and hip.

On the day we went for the X-ray, Frankie was excited – at the prospect of missing a day from school, and of seeing the inside of a general hospital. She was fascinated by medical matters, and I remember her exclaiming gleefully, as we sat waiting for the X-ray: 'Isn't it *interesting*, Mummy?'

It was a phrase which was often on her lips, for I suppose she had what is commonly described as an 'inquiring mind'. She was always asking questions – sometimes most embarrassing ones! There was an openness and a vivacity about her which suffered no inhibitions, and which often expressed itself in a warm demonstrativeness which brought the two of us – her and me – particularly close.

We were two of a kind, and, as so often happens in families, we tended to develop a special understanding for one another, while Elizabeth's temperament matched up better with Arthur's.

Elizabeth, with her long blonde hair and almost classic features, was more reserved than her sister, though very sweet-natured. She spent a good deal of her time on a neighbouring farm with a friend, for she loved the outdoor life. Frankie, however, was really far happier running about the village with younger children, and was in many ways a 'homebird'. In this contrast of temperament and interests we were later to see so clearly the hand of God.

One really warm May day, when Frankie was fishing for

newts in the village pond with her friends, I had to take a quick trip into Haywards Heath, our nearest town two miles away. It was a Saturday afternoon, and as the bus I was in passed the pond, I caught sight of Frankie's little figure in her red tartan trews and blue jersey, her short blonde hair shining in the sunlight.

The memory of her is stamped indelibly on my heart, for it was the last time I was to look at her without either the fear or the knowledge that she was seriously ill.

She was so intent with her fishing net, that she didn't see me waving from the bus, but when I came back, she was still there by the pond and this time she did see me. She came running up to the bus-stop, greeted me with her impish smile, took my hand and walked home with me.

'Tired of newting?' I asked.

She shook her head. 'No, but my leg hurts badly. And I've got a wet foot.'

This she said quite calmly, and with the smile still lighting up her blue eyes. I gave her some clean socks, wondering if the trouble could be rheumatism. The X-rays had shown nothing.

Frankie lay back in a deck chair, humming to herself for a while. Then:

'Mummy, why do you think my leg hurts if there's nothing wrong with it?'

'Darling, I wish I knew.'

She got up and hopped around the garden.

'Don't do that, dear. You must exercise it – try to walk normally. Without the limp. Let me see if you can do it.'

She put the foot down gingerly, and immediately lifted it up with a little gasp of pain.

'I can't, Mummy. I can't even put it down on the ground.'

By now, as can be imagined, I was feeling really worried. I knew now that this was not just a question of 'nerves' – that there was no pretence about the limp she had developed of late. During the week-end, things got progressively worse

There was no cheerful smile now – Frankie was in real and intense pain.

'Do something, Mummy,' she pleaded. 'It hurts terribly. It's an awful jabbing pain . . . ohhh!'

But the doctor was still completely baffled. Each time he called he repeated his original diagnosis of either 'growing pains' or 'nerves'. He said he could find nothing whatsoever wrong with the leg or the hip, and that the X-ray had confirmed this. As Frankie usually seemed to be having a comparatively peaceful spell when he arrived, and therefore greeted him with her usual wide smile, he could not be expected to understand how severe the pain was.

We tried all the creams and lotions we could find, but the pain only grew worse. Day and night it continued, until we were all exhausted with worry and fatigue.

Now, Frankie would only let her Daddy touch the leg – she said he had a way of rubbing it which was better than anyone else's touch. She would say:

'Be careful with me, Daddy. Please be careful . . .'

'I will, sweetheart. I'll be as careful as I can.'

That afternoon when Frankie and I were alone (Arthur carried her downstairs each day and put her on the sofa), she suddenly said:

'Mummy, if Jesus were here, He would only have to walk into this room and touch me and this awful pain would be gone.'

'Darling, Jesus can make that leg better, even though He isn't on earth any more. He's alive, although we can't see Him.'

'Well then, let's ask Him to do it!' She looked at me as if to say, 'What are we waiting for?'

So we prayed that Jesus would make the leg better. But when we had finished, an extra hard jab of pain came, and after a while Frankie said:

'Why did Jesus make my leg hurt in the first place, Mummy?'

I tried to explain that it wasn't Jesus who was making her leg hurt, but repeated that He could make it better, if we really believed.

'Why doesn't He then?' she demanded. 'I believe He can. Why does He let it go on hurting me?'

What does a mother say when a child asks questions like this? Misery and anxiety blurred my thoughts.

That night, as I lay in Frankie's bed – she was sleeping with Arthur, in order that Elizabeth and I might get a little sleep – I pleaded with God that He would show us what to do. During that night the pain was so intense that neither Arthur nor Frankie had any sleep. In the morning, after I had lifted her back into her own bed, I went back into our bedroom to ask Arthur what kind of night they had had.

To my dismay, he broke down completely.

'She's such a little thing,' was all he could say. 'She looked so tiny and frail, lying there, and I felt so helpless . . .'

Later, he told me that in the night, in desperation, he had laid his hands on Frankie and prayed that God would heal her. Neither of us had thought very much about the question of healing up till now – we had had no cause to. But to our relief and amazement, Frankie now told us that the pain had gone.

We kept her lying on the bed during the morning because the doctor had promised to call in, but she was like a different child. She talked cheerfully, even saying that she fancied some cauliflower cheese for dinner. All the week she had eaten practically nothing, except a few nibbles of bread and butter. When Arthur came in at midday, he was overjoyed to see that she was still free from pain. It was then that he told me how he had 'laid his hands' on her in the night.

I would emphasize here that we believe Frankie never again *consciously* experienced pain of the intense nature that she had suffered during that week – except for a brief bout which she had just as the doctor arrived that same afternoon. But this particular attack we always considered to be necessary in order that the doctor might actually see how severe and real it was. He had not actually seen her in the grip of the pain before. But now, he said at once that Frankie must go to hospital, where routine tests could be made, so that some explanation might be found for the mysterious symptoms which had hitherto baffled him completely.

When she knew that she was to go to hospital, Frankie was inconsolable. She begged and pleaded that we would not let her go, and in spite of all my encouraging descriptions of what it would be like, and of how she would enjoy it, she could only remember that I had said all that before on a previous occasion, when she had gone into an isolation hospital with scarlet-fever in London, and found herself to be the only child there.

Eventually, assuring her that this time it would really be different, and that she would be in a children's ward with others of her own age, she stopped crying and allowed herself to be carried into the waiting ambulance. As she was being lifted in, a group of small children gathered to watch on their way home from school.

'What's the matter with Frankie?' they chorused. 'Why are they putting her in there?'

How can I describe my feelings as I said good-bye to Arthur, watched him kiss Frankie, then settled down in the ambulance for the short three-mile trip to the hospital? Any mother who has taken an ailing child to hospital will know something of the sick dread and misery. But after the strain of the past week, real panic and terror now held me in its grip. What could be wrong with my precious child? Could it be polio, or some other form of crippling or even fatal paralysis? I bit my lips to keep back the tears: whatever happened I must not break down now . . .

Then, cautiously, I glanced at Frankie, as she lay wrapped in a red blanket on the stretcher. To my amazement the tear-stained little face broke into a radiant smile.

Later, I asked her why she had smiled at me like that, when

only a few minutes earlier she had been so unhappy and afraid.

'Well, you see,' she answered, 'it was because I knew you were nearly crying with worry about me, and I smiled to make you happy, because I love you so much.'

This was typical of the selfless courage with which she faced the long period of illness which was to follow. And courage in a little child can be more heartbreaking than self-pity or complaining. So we were to find.

I should mention that at this time she was nine years old, and Elizabeth nearly twelve.

Chapter 4

The weeks which followed were full of uneasiness for Arthur and myself. Every day one or other of us visited the hospital, and although Frankie was still in no pain, she seemed to be slipping into a very low condition. Her regular question: 'When can I come home?' I had to meet with a vague 'When the doctor says you are well enough, darling'.

We were now told that arthritis was probably the cause of the trouble, but as the weeks went by and this diagnosis was neither confirmed nor refuted, our anxiety grew. One day I buttonholed a young houseman who came into the ward to take a specimen of blood. (This was being done twice a week at the time.)

'*Is* it arthritis?' I challenged him. 'Only it seems to me that nobody is absolutely certain.'

'As a matter of fact,' he replied, 'we're not certain. That's why we keep making these tests. You see, Frances has a very low blood count – there is a steady drop in the number of white cells, and this may mean a number of things . . .'

I watched him walk off down the corridor, his white coat swinging, and the full meaning of what he had said broke over me like a cold sea wave. *A low blood count . . . This may mean a number of things . . .* Suddenly, I wanted to run after the retreating form of the cheerful young houseman and ask the question which now burned in my mind: *'Could it possibly be leukaemia?'*

Instead, I stood there by the bed, struggling to hide my terror from Frankie's searching, but weary gaze.

One day, when Frankie had been in hospital for nearly

four weeks, I arrived to find her in a very deep sleep. Sister explained that one final test had been made on her – a test made under a sedative.

'If it proves negative,' she said, 'then we shall go ahead and treat for arthritis.'

'What kind of test?' I asked.

Sister hesitated. 'We have taken some . . . fluid . . . from her chest. The results will be several days coming through.'

Each day, as we waited for the result of the mysterious 'test', the suspense grew. But at the same time, we were becoming more and more conscious of the deep peace of God in our hearts. As we travelled to and fro on the buses, through the lovely Sussex countryside; as we walked through the meadows which formed a short cut from the bus-stop to the hospital, gazing across the burnished gold of the butter-cup filled fields to the distant downs, blue and blurred in the summer haze; or as we lay in bed at night with our minds on that frail little form who might, or might not be sleeping peacefully at that moment in her narrow hospital bed – as we did all these things, a quiet voice seemed to be constantly penetrating our restless thoughts:

'*Thou wilt keep him in perfect peace,*' whispered the Voice, '*whose mind is stayed on thee, because he trusteth in thee . . .*'

Never, at any time during this grave trial, did we have any difficulty in sleeping at night. This was one of the wonders which never ceased to amaze us and others – a sign of the depth of the 'peace' which was indeed ours. Often, during this time, as I fell asleep the words: 'And so He giveth His beloved sleep' . . . would drift across my fading consciousness. We proved that His peace is not something which touches only the surface of the mind: it penetrates to the very depth of one's being.

I think that Arthur and I both knew that something tremendous was about to happen to us. It was as though we were waiting, hand in hand, outside a locked door. . . . Figures came and went, unlocking the door and slipping inside, or appearing suddenly from the other side of it, hurrying past us with averted eyes, but always taking care to lock the door behind them. . . .

At the same time, we had no real fear of what lay beyond the locked door. We anticipated no darkness or terror. It was only in the faces of others, the ones who were constantly passing in and out, that we saw anything that might make us afraid. And it was the waiting which was so hard to bear . . .

One morning during this waiting period, Frankie said to me:

'Mummy, last night when the night-nurses came on duty, I heard one of them say to the other: 'This little girl is very ill. Her blood count is getting lower and lower.' I expect they thought I was asleep. . . . What did they mean, Mummy? *Am* I very ill?'

When I asked if Frankie could have some fruit I had brought her, the Sister replied quietly: 'She can have just anything she fancies, Mrs. Mitson. Anything.'

'Why do you say that? Isn't she eating still?'

The Sister turned her head and looked out of the window.

'She is eating hardly anything at all.'

This was on a Saturday. Sister told me that if I could be at the hospital fairly early on Monday morning, I could see the Specialist, who would give me the result of the test they had made.

The Sunday after was a memorable one. Arthur preached in the morning from the story of Nehemiah. He was doing a series at the time, and on this particular day his sermon title was 'Prepared for the Task'.

To preach two sermons a week and conduct a Sunday School, when your child is lying in hospital with a strange undiagnosed disease is no easy matter. Each week I marvelled that Arthur could stand up in the pulpit and preach with such freedom and power. I marvelled that his finely strung nervous system could stand up to this kind of emotional strain. The answer is, of course, that the strength and courage he showed in those days, and in the long days which were to follow, were not his own. If they had been, they would have surely failed him.

Arthur preached that morning on the preparation of Nehemiah for the task of the rebuilding of the walls of Jerusalem. He pointed out that God prepares us for the tasks He gives us to do in life. Sometimes the preparation begins way back in childhood; often it goes back even farther than that, when heredity or character or temperament are to play an important part in God's purpose for a life. All the time, through the seemingly unimportant periods of our lives, through the most ordinary, or maybe the most extraordinary and baffling circumstances, God prepares us for His purposes.

Vaguely, I felt that this message was for me.

That evening after church, we were listening to part of Handel's 'Messiah' played on our record-player. Usually on a Sunday evening there was somebody in for coffee, and I don't think we were alone on this particular evening. Sitting there with my eyes closed, listening to the music, I was in that kind of no-man's-land of the mind when one is partially following a train of thought, and partially conscious of other, outside influences which claim one's attention and demand something of one's inner senses.

Various pictures were passing before my mind: Frankie being wheeled about the village in a wheelchair; Frankie grown up, but still in a wheelchair – stunted perhaps, but still with the same round smiling face and shining blue eyes. I had always been terrified of having to nurse anyone for a prolonged period. It was one of the things which I believed God would never ask of me, knowing, as He did, how utterly useless I would be. . . .

I cannot now remember at which particular point it was during the playing of those records, whether it was during a vocal rendering, or during the trumpet solo, or at the height of one of the magnificent choruses. But all at once, the stirrings, the mental pictures, the thoughts, the tangle of emotions within me seemed to shift, to assemble themselves together, to take shape.

And out of that moment there emerged a single, piercing beam of light, which shook me, without warning into a blinding awareness of my immediate surroundings – the faded red carpet, the brighter red of the record-player, the gleaming rows of many-coloured books which lined the walls, the fluorescent green of the apple tree outside the window. . . .

Out of this heightened awareness, breathtaking in its sharpness and simplicity, came this knowledge: that whatever lay behind the locked door of tomorrow, whatever suffering or grief, or hardship or trial, whatever sacrifice, whatever toil, whatever task – whatever making or breaking – then, by the grace of God, I was ready for it: prepared for the task. . . . As soon as the door was unlocked, then I would pass through it – not with resignation, nor with mere acceptance, or even with trembling faith, *but with joy*.

The room remained unchanged, the music continued to play, and the other figures in the room still sat listening, immobile. But for me, the summer twilight was aflame with a quiet radiance.

Chapter 5

Monday morning dawned bright and sunny. When Arthur asked me whether he should go with me to the hospital that morning, or whether I would be happy to go alone, I replied that I didn't think there was any need for him to come. After all, I said, it was only a question of having a word with the Specialist, and probably of having the original diagnosis confirmed. If, by any chance, the Specialist was unable to confirm this diagnosis and there was something new to reveal, then I would ring Arthur from the hospital immediately. In any case, he would be visiting Frankie that afternoon.

On my way to the hospital, the word 'prepared' kept repeating itself in my mind. This sense of 'preparedness' was so strong that I felt it must be almost tangible. Echoing the words of St. Paul, in J. B. Phillip's rendering, I thought with wonder: 'I am ready for anything, through the strength of the One who lives within me.'

Ready for anything? *Anything?* Even—? I put the grim thought quickly from me. This day of golden summer was surely not the time for such morbid imaginings.. And after all, few diseases these days were fatal. Except, of course . . . And *that,* so my mind argued, had been ruled out already. So I put the thought from me; but not before, somewhere, deep down in my most secret innermost spirit, a voice had gasped: *'Yes, ready, even for the ultimate sorrow – in His strength!'*

Frankie was bright and happy that morning when I arrived. Perhaps it was the thought that the Specialist, who alone had the authority to say she could go home, was coming in to see her. Perhaps it was simply that the sun was shining and I had arrived early. But I was pleased to see that she was sitting up with her hair nicely combed, and a clean, wild-rose-patterned nightie tied neatly under her chin with a big pink ribbon.

Glancing round the ward, I was struck by the sad sophistication of some of the other children. Peter, a boy of thirteen, was engaged in a suggestive kind of backchat with one of the orderlies; Betty, who was two years younger than Frankie, was studying the pages of a teen-age magazine; a new girl whom I had not seen before, with horn-rimmed glasses and a sallow complexion, had her ear glued to a transistor radio. The unmistakable nasal wail of the Beatles filled the ward, and on one of the walls there were pin-ups of various show personalities.

Among all this, I couldn't help thinking, rather sentimentally, that Frankie looked like a little dew-pearled English hedge-rose, as she sat there doing a jig-saw, and watching the door eagerly for my arrival.

She leaned towards me confidentially when I had pulled up a chair by her bed.

'See that new girl with the glasses? Her language is awful! I asked her if she went to Sunday School, and, of course, she doesn't. I suggested she tries it when she gets out of hospital!' Then, in a different voice: 'Do you think the doctor will let me come home, Mummy? Do you think he will? Do you know, I've been here nearly five weeks?'

The doctor was late doing his rounds that morning. When, finally, word came that he was 'on the way', I went out into the corridor and walked down as far as the fish-tank. My heart beat frantically as I watched the three white-coated figures pause outside the ward to examine the notes Sister had ready; then pushing open the swing doors, they went inside.

I fixed my eyes on the cheerful grin of the angel fish, as he darted to and fro in the brightly lit tank, but soon I was clutching my stomach to stop the lurching sensation which was increasing there. A nurse came out of the sluice and smiled at me.

'I've got butterflies, nurse,' I told her with a forced grin.

'Butterflies? Is it you they're doing in there, then?'

'No,' I replied, 'but it's a little bit of me!'

After what seemed like an eternity, the swing doors of the ward opened outwards, and the three white-coated figures appeared again. Once more, they stopped to peruse the notes, talking in undertones, gesticulating, rubbing their chins. I caught such phrases as 'most difficult', 'early diagnosis', 'puzzling factors' . . . I knew instinctively, that they were discussing Frankie's case.

At last, they began to walk slowly down the corridor towards me, the Specialist leading the way, the two housemen bringing up the rear. Quickly I stood up, and as they drew level, I searched their faces frantically for some sign of what they were about to say. None of them smiled.

'Now, Mrs. Mitson.' It was the Specialist speaking. 'Would you like to come into Sister's office for a moment?'

He held the door for me, and I went in, a kind of deadly calm now holding me in its grip. To my surprise, all three doctors followed me into the little room and shut the door behind them. The Specialist sat down in Sister's chair, and picked up some papers on the desk. He motioned me to sit down on a chair opposite. The other doctors, who seemed to be staring at a point just beyond their toes, remained standing. The atmosphere in the room was electric.

'Now, Mrs. Mitson.' (Eyes lowered behind horn-rimmed spectacles. Sensitive fingers perfectly still on the desk) . . . 'As you know, we have been rather puzzled by Frances's symptoms. There have been a number of things which somehow didn't seem to fit in.'

He lifted his head and looked at me, and I nodded, passing a hot tongue over my dry lips.

'But finally, we decided to give Frances a rather special test, and now that the result has come through, I am afraid that I have some rather serious news for you.'

Still, from the top of my head to the tip of my toes, I was aware of a deadly calm, as though the very blood in my veins had congealed and rendered me insensible. Dimly I was aware that the gaze of the two standing housemen had lifted, that they were now watching me with defensive, clinical caution. I kept my eyes fixed on the lips of the Specialist, waiting for the next words to come.

'I am afraid she has a very serious bone disease. . . .'

A sharp splinter of ice spiralled downwards from somewhere at the back of my throat. Somewhere, in the darkest caverns of my mind a hoarse whisper echoed: *If you sit perfectly still and do not even breathe, the next moment need never come . . .*

'She has leukaemia.'

Now the eyes of all three men fixed on me guardedly. Did they expect me to scream? To faint? To fall off the chair at their feet? To burst into uncontrollable hysterics? For a moment the room, the white-coated doctors, the narrow window which looked out on to a green lawn, were petrified into a kind of stone tableau. No one stirred. Then I heard my own voice say quietly: 'I see.'

The housemen shifted their weight from one foot to the other. The Specialist said quickly: 'I am very sorry.'

I looked at his shoes and thought how small his feet were. I looked at his hands and saw them moving ineffectually among the papers on the desk. I looked at his face and thought: 'What a ghastly task for him . . . what a ghastly thing to have to tell a mother . . .'

I said, pressing my fingernails into the palm of my hand: 'There isn't anything you can do for that, is there?' My voice was low, but calm.

For some reason, this seemed to ease the tension in the room. Everybody shifted.

'Oh, yes!' exclaimed the Specialist, grateful, I thought, that

I had asked a question to which he could give a positive answer. 'There are many things we can do, and we shall begin right away. We have some wonderful drugs which we can give – in fact, in a day or two Frances will be feeling really fit – better, maybe, than she has felt for years —'

I cut him short.

'But the effect will be only temporary, won't it? I mean, in the end . . . nothing will be any good . . . will it?'

Tension returned to the room again. One of the housemen coughed uneasily.

I said: 'Doctor, tell me. How long will it be? How long before — ?'

He leaned back in his chair and looked at me now with unmasked compassion.

'Six months . . . a year . . .' he leaned forward again and picked up his pen, not looking at me now, and added quickly: 'Maybe even two years. And in the meantime, who knows what might come up? We're working on this thing, you know, all the time. We're —'

But I turned away from him now and stared out of the window, grief and horror sweeping over me at last, like a cold, dark tide. *Six months. A year. Two years!* Had he said that Frankie could not last the week, that it was only a matter of days, then I felt I could have borne it. But this! It was more than any mother could bear! The slow torture, the waiting and watching, the concealments; I had read enough about the disease to know a little of what was in store. . . . Desperately I slammed the door of my mind against the torrent of thoughts and emotions which converged upon it from all directions.

I stood up. From far away, I heard my voice ask:

'When can I have her home, doctor?'

Again, he seemed grateful for a question which did not require an evasive answer.

'As soon as we can possibly manage it,' he said brightly. 'Let me see, treatment will start today, and in a day or so she should be strong enough to walk about the ward. Then in about a week or ten days, you can take her home.'

I reached for the door-handle, and the two housemen leaped to open the door for me.

Turning back towards the Specialist, I said quietly:

'Thank you, doctor.'

Then I was out in the corridor again. The angel fish grinned at me as I passed his tank. There was no one else in sight. A dozen or more steps and I would be in the ward, standing by Frankie's bed . . .

I stopped, summoning all my strength to sweep clear my mind of all thought, to drain my heart dry of all emotion, to calm my trembling body into stillness. For in a matter of seconds I must face my innocent, condemned child, my little wild rose, and answer her eager question: 'What did he say, Mummy? Can I come home?'

I pushed open the door of the ward and went in.

Immediately the wide blue eyes met mine, searching, pleading:

'Can I come home? Is it arthritis? What did he say?'

I smiled. Dear God, how did I do it? I smiled. Then I said:

'You're coming home in a week, darling. Just think of it, only one more week. And he says you can get out of bed in a day or two and walk about the ward. Isn't that marvellous?'

'You look kind of funny.'

'Do I, pet? Well, maybe I'm a bit tired . . . Now look. Your dinner's just coming, and I've got to ring Daddy. I'm going to ask him to come over, and then he and I can get a bit to eat in the village, and then come back and spend all the afternoon with you. How's that?'

'All right, but don't be long. . . . Gosh, I can hardly believe I'm coming home at last! Maybe Sister'll let me get out of this old bed today. Do you think she will?'

I crossed the tarmac towards the telephone kiosk, constricting myself carefully within the rigid bounds of control which I knew I must hold, now, for the rest of the day. One minute at a time . . . That was essential . . . One moment at a time, from this moment on. Don't think, don't feel, don't let up for a minute. If you do you're finished . . .

I dialled our home number and stood listening to the sound of the bell ringing. Then Arthur's voice said: 'Hullo' – breathlessly, in my ear.

'Darling, are you ready for a shock?' No good beating about the bush.

Immediately, he replied: 'Yes, I'm ready.'

And I knew, with gratitude, that he was.

'It's leukaemia.'

From the other end of the line, a strangled sound, but no word.

Then: 'How long?'

'He said six months, a year, maybe even two . . . Oh, Arthur, I feel that if he had said she couldn't see the week out, I could have borne it . . .'

'The Lord knows all about it, sweetheart . . Maybe He'll take her soon. . . .'

'Arthur?'

'Yes?'

'Can you come, darling? Right away?'

I was crying now, and I dabbed furiously at the tears, steeling myself to remember that from this moment only one thing mattered. Frankie herself must never, must never guess. Not by a word, or a gesture, a sigh or a tear must she ever know the secret which we must lock in our hearts.

I stumbled out of the kiosk, and stood there a moment in the hot June sunshine. All around me, things were going on as before. A car pulled into the car park, a white-coated porter wheeled a trolley towards out-patients, a group of nurses crossed chattering and laughing from the dining hall. . . .

I felt that I was somehow projected outside myself, looking on, with a kind of frozen indifference, at the plump figure which was me; a woman in her early thirties in a pink and white gingham suit, fair hair framing a face that stared blankly across the courtyard. An awful sense of alone-ness enveloped me. I was untouchable, unreachable, in my brittle tower of transparent ice.

Then, as I stared at the group of nurses who strolled, red-lined cloaks hanging casually from their shoulders, on their way to lunch, one of the figures grew oddly familiar before my eyes. I stared for a moment in disbelief, then, at the top of my voice I shouted:

'Coral!'

She turned immediately, and saw me standing there. For some reason I didn't move, but stayed there and waited for her to come to me. I knew, of course, that Coral was working at the hospital, but not once, during the whole of the long period when I had been visiting Frankie daily, had I ever run into her by chance like this. Yet at that very moment, in my crucial hour of need, she had walked into my line of vision.

She took one look at my face, then asked quickly:

'How's Frances?'

I put my arms round her and told her.

As she led me over to the ward where she had worked part-time since Ray's death, she murmured: 'What can I say to you? What can I say?'

'Don't say anything, please . . .'

But she said gently: 'It'll break your heart, Eileen, but the Lord will carry you through. He'll give you a strength you never dreamed of. And have you thought? – they'll know each other in heaven? . . .'

But I didn't want to think about heaven. I wasn't ready for that yet. It was no comfort for me think of Frankie in heaven. What did we really know of that other life, anyway? The thought of eternal joys were of little consolation when all one's poor, finite mind could long for was to be allowed to go on living this imperfect, earthly life in the same way as one had lived it yesterday. 'Safe in the arms of Jesus' meant nothing when all I wanted, or she wanted, was to be safe in the arms of each other . . .

I sat on the laundry basket in the corridor of Coral's ward and drank the tea she gave me. Then, slowly, I made my way towards the village to meet Arthur. Sitting on the wooden bench in the High Street waiting for his bus to pull in, I thought:

'My poor, sensitive Arthur . . . How is he going to bear this? What will happen now? Who will preach for him next Sunday – and all the other Sundays? How can he possibly carry on?'

The bus arrived, and the next moment he was beside me on the seat. As soon as we touched each other, our control broke. He told me afterwards that he had not shed a tear until he saw me sitting there. Now we sat locked in each other's arms there by the busy main road, oblivious of curious passers-by, and of the constant stream of traffic which passed up and down the street. People turned and stared out of cars and lorries and buses, as there we sat, imprisoned in our private world of unspeakable grief, and wept. After a while, I managed to say:

'How will you carry on, darling? What will you do?'

'What will *I* do?' He burst into fresh tears. 'What about you, sweetheart, what about *you*?'

It was this recognition of our love for each other, a love which was concerned, even at a time like this, primarily with the need of the other, which steadied us both in that agonizing moment. We dried our eyes, brushed ourselves down, smiled shakily at each other, and began to walk slowly down the street, our hands still firmly clasped.

Neither of us felt like eating, but we had an hour before Frankie would expect us back in the ward. A precious hour in which to muster all the strength and control we would need, and to draw deeply upon those inner spiritual resources which we knew, even in that black hour, could not fail us.

Ironically, the only place we could find to sit in privacy was the churchyard. As we approached the lovely old gateway, the magnificent vista of blue downland was framed as usual by the ancient arch, but today its beauty was lost upon us. We passed under the arch and walked through the graveyard to a quiet seat overlooking the rolling landscape beyond.

A year or so before, we had sat in this very same spot – all four of us – and ate a picnic lunch. Now, I remembered, with cruel clarity, how Frankie had wandered, fascinated, among the tombstones, reading the inscriptions aloud.

'Look, Mummy, there's one like a swiss roll! And look, a whole family's buried here! And here's one belonging to a girl of eight – gosh, the same age as me!'

When, finally, we made our way back to the hospital, our stomachs were sick with dread. How were we going to sit there, by her bed, all the afternoon without giving something away? She was so quick to notice the smallest thing – so sensitive to the feelings of others. I could not bear the thought of deceiving her, when the two of us had always been so close, so open with each other, so spontaneous. . . . I pleaded with God to give us all that we needed.

The first thing she said was: 'Daddy, you're tired. And Mummy still looks a bit funny to me. You'd better both get an early night! Isn't it marvellous, Daddy? I can come home in a week. And Sister said tomorrow I can get out of bed and sit in the wheelchair, and then next day you can wheel me round the grounds!'

She chattered on brightly, and a passing nurse stopped to smile at her. Looking from Frankie's face then back to mine, she said: 'My, isn't she like her Mummy?'

Quickly, Arthur turned his head away so that he shouldn't have to see the stark truth in those innocently spoken words. Knowing that he was struggling for control, I widened my already impossible smile, as Frankie leaned forward and rubbed her nose playfully on mine, pleased at what the nurse had said.

'I forget how long we sat there talking and laughing

together, but I remember the awful mixture of relief and dismay with which my control broke as soon as we were clear of the hospital.

Elizabeth's first question when she came in from school was, as usual: 'How's Frankie?'

She looked from Arthur's face to mine with alarmed suspicion.

'She's coming home next week!' I said cheerfully, only too conscious of my red, swollen eyes and nose.

'Then why have you been crying?' she asked sharply.

Elizabeth was twelve. Too young to be told the truth, too old to be content with half-truths. Yet this latter course, I knew, was the only one open to us at this moment.

'Oh well,' we said, 'you know how worried we've all been . . . The strain has got just a little too much today.'

'*Is* it arthritis?'

I remembered how Frankie had asked that question earlier the same day. I hadn't given a direct answer, and she hadn't bothered to pursue it, for all she really cared about was coming home. This wouldn't do for Elizabeth.

'No,' I said, cutting bread and butter vigorously. 'It's not arthritis. The doctor says Frankie has something wrong with her blood. It's a rare illness, but they're going to give her some special drugs . . .'

'That's all right, then, isn't it?'

'Yes, dear. That's all right . . .'

That evening, when Elizabeth had gone off down to the farm, Arthur and I were once more alone with our nightmare secret. We found that we could not sit in the house. Claustrophobic horror closed in on us when we tried.

We went out into the garden and stood under the apple tree. *But here was where I had sat that afternoon when she had hopped around on one leg in her red trews . . .*

We crossed over to the rabbit hutch. The innocent furry animals looked up at us from their round, fawn eyes. The white baby with the brown ears was for Frankie, but she had not seen it yet. . . . *'I can't wait to see the rabbits, Mummy – especially mine!*

I turned away from them, and buried my face in Arthur's coat. As his arms came round me, and our salty, tear-wet lips met in a desperate kiss, I thought: *'This was how she began . . . the darling fruit of our love!'*

She was everywhere. There was no way to turn. Every possible escape route was blocked with the inexorable truth.

Chapter 6

The terror lasted only for a moment. By the middle of the evening, the hidden strength of God, which we had known from the outset would never fail us, was beginning to rise again in our wounded spirits like an amaranthine flower. Slowly we became aware of a strange calm filling our minds.

Arthur had already telephoned around to cancel our speaking engagements for the week (I had had one for that very evening), and one of the calls had been taken by the daughter of one of our ministerial friends who lived several miles away. Now, as we sat talking of practical things – how much to tell Elizabeth, whether to keep this thing a secret from the village, etc., a knock suddenly sounded at the door. The next moment, Arthur was showing our friends into the room.

As they embraced us, wept with us, prayed with us, the whole situation continued to change before our eyes. Like lights going on one by one in a dark room, so the words of faith and comfort which passed to and fro between us began gradually to illumine the darkness of our hearts.

'Prepared for the task' . . . Wasn't this how it was with us? And what was the task? Could we be sure that the dreaded end we had been told to expect was what God had in store for us? Did we not believe that God was more powerful than this thing? That He could step in and save our darling from death if such was His perfect will? Excitement, challenge, the glorious certainty of God's sovereignty and power now filled our horizon.

God had chosen us for a task of terrifying proportions. Ours to discover the nature of that task, and then to carry it through in His strength. But underlying all our thoughts was the awesome knowledge of complete submission to His will. We were entirely and unconditionally in His hands.

Among the messages of sympathy which poured into our house during the next few days (giving us, at times, a sense of unreality, as though Frankie were already dead) came this simple reminder: 'It is not a question of struggling for faith, but of knowing peace through surrender.'

Surrender. This, we knew, was the most important thing of all. God could heal – the power of His Son Jesus Christ was the same yesterday, today and forever. But before we dare ask for such a tremendous thing, we must surrender ourselves without reserve to His purposes, whatever they might be.

In talking to Sister a few days after the diagnosis was made, I found that she, too, shared our faith in the greatness of God.

'Of course He can heal,' she said. 'How can we doubt that? But don't pin all you have on that hope. I have seen this happen before – with disastrous results.'

Quietly, I replied: 'We shan't do that, Sister. By the grace of God, we have already accepted whatever God has in store for us.'

'Then you will be all right,' was her reply.

How can I explain the transformation which took place in our hearts and minds during these days? On the Sunday after we had been told of the tragic news, Arthur was in his usual place in the pulpit, and the sermon he preached was entitled: 'The Greatness of God.' He, who could be broken down emotionally by far lesser things, nevertheless stood erect and unwavering in the pulpit that Sunday morning while the sentence of death lay upon his little daughter.

'"Hast thou not known?"' he quoted, '"Hast thou not heard, that the everlasting God, the Lord, the Creator of the ends of the earth fainteth not, neither is weary? There is no searching of His understanding . . ."

'Everything human is subject to change and decay. Our

great buildings crumble and fall; the *Titanic* went out as an unsinkable ship, but was utterly destroyed; the League of Nations, after the First World War, was set up to end all war – but what happened? And man, with all his pride and progress, cannot prolong life. . . .

'But God is everlasting. . . . He is Lord of all. God is still on the throne – and He will remember His own. Do you really believe that God has everything under His control? The international situation? The national situation? The personal situation? . . .

'God is working His sovereign purposes out in the affairs of men. The fundamental question is: "Is He *my* Lord? Is God *my* God?" God was in Christ, reconciling the world unto Himself. . . . God hath given to us eternal life, and this life in His Son. If you have Him, you have all you need and more beside. When you are losing your grip, exhausted with anxiety, burdened beyond endurance – when all earthly props have gone: *then He gives strength.* "They that wait upon the Lord shall renew their strength, they shall mount up with wings, as eagles . . ."

'Oh, wait upon Him! Be utterly dependent upon Him! Let go – and let God!'

Let go and let God . . . This was our experience during those days, and the days which were to follow. In letting go, we allowed ourselves to be lifted up above the darkness and hopelessness of the human situation in which we found ourselves; lifted up above the dark clouds, into the glory of God's sunlight; lifted up, borne up, as if on eagles' wings . . .

We decided, that in order that God might be glorified, we should not keep our secret from the village, even if we could. We believed that now, in our extremity, was God's opportunity to show Himself to those around us. All eyes were upon us.

The whole village was stricken when news of Frankie's illness became known. Some people broke down in the street when they asked after her, and we had to tell them the news.

We found that people we did not ourselves know by name, knew Frankie – 'the little girl with the lovely smile'.

As Arthur and I went about our work with a calm serenity, people looked at us in astonishment. Folk who were afraid to meet us face to face because of our grief, soon found they had nothing to fear in this. Quietly, we told all who questioned our peace of mind, that God would carry us through.

At the hospital, as we visited Frankie during those last days of her stay there, none of the other visiting mothers had any idea of what was wrong with her. When, just before we took her home, I told one of the mothers whom I had got to know quite well, she was dumbfounded.

'But you seem so happy!' she exclaimed. 'I've been watching you these last few days, and I thought you must have had some wonderful news, you were so radiant. How can you be like that?'

So I told her of the faith we had in God, and of the prayers which were ascending to heaven daily from all our friends on our behalf. She turned away embarrassed, but I knew she would not forget.

And as the news spread far and wide among our friends, so the volume of prayer for us increased, and so the wonderful sense of the power and presence of God grew stronger each day.

One evening I was given a lift home in the car of the hospital medical technologist, who lived in the same village, and whose daughter was in the same form at school as Frankie. As we drove home together, I ventured to say:

'You know, of course, what's wrong with Frankie?'

He was silent for a moment, before saying quietly:

'I found it.'

It had not occurred to me before that this would be so. I knew the position that Mr. Hood held at the hospital, but still I had never actually pictured him taking that fatal drop of bone marrow that had been extracted from Frankie's breastbone on that day I had found her sedated, and himself putting it under his microscope, and seeing with his own eyes that ghastly evidence of disease. Now it was my turn to be silent. After a while, Mr. Hood spoke again.

'I'm sorry,' he said, 'that I kept you waiting so long for the result. But to be quite honest with you, I took one look and put it aside for a day before I could bear to look again.'

'Please don't apologise,' I said. 'If you had had the result through by the Friday instead of the Monday, we would have had the week-end to live through. My husband would never have been able, by the Sunday, to get up in the pulpit and preach two sermons. As it was, he had nearly a week's grace.'

He looked at me sideways.

'You've made me feel a whole lot better,' he said.

As I got out of the car, he went on: 'Don't forget, if there's anything – absolutely anything – we can do for Frankie, just let us know. Nothing will be too much trouble. She'll be needing pretty frequent blood-tests once she's out of hospital. Don't trail up there every time – just give me a ring and I'll be right round and do the job myself.'

Mr. Hood's kindness was one of the many blessings we were to experience during the coming year. Frankie loved him, and the fact that he was her school-friend's Dad did a great deal to make the whole unpleasant business of blood-tests, and the occasional sternum-marrow test, almost a routine thing. When grown men sat in the path. lab. and trembled at the prospect of that probing needle which was to draw blood from their veins, Mr. Hood would quote the case of a little girl he knew who had the same kind of needle in her arm every week of her life (sometimes twice a week) – and never made a murmur.

On the mornings when he was due to come for some blood, Frankie would sit up in bed grinning, and as he sat on the side of the bed and showed her how to pump up the vein ready for the needle, he would laugh and joke with her, tell her what his daughter Liz had been doing that morning, and end up by remarking that, of course, the reason why he was always able to fill his little phial with blood so easily was entirely due to the cleverness and skill of the patient!

Sometimes, towards the end of the illness, when Frankie could not manage to smile, and had hardly the strength to pump her fingers into the palm of her hand to raise the vein, he would sit on the bed and look at her with the same grin and the same bantering talk. No one would have guessed how deeply his heart grieved, or how much he dreaded making the inevitable blood count when he returned to the path. lab.

Though Mr. Hood might be surprised to hear me say so, we always regarded him as one of God's direct gifts to us during those uphill weeks and months.

It was to Mr. Hood that I eventually put the question which had been puzzling me for some time. Why, if leukaemia was an abnormal multiplication of the white cells, had I been told that the number of Frankie's white blood cells were dropping drastically? Mr. Hood explained that Frankie had a slightly more unusual type of disease which should, strictly speaking, be known as 'aleukaemic leukaemia'. In other words, the cancer cells in the bone marrow destroyed the white cells in her case, instead of causing them to multiply.

'Is this a more serious type of leukaemia?' I asked him.

'Not more serious,' he said. 'Just a different picture. But in all cases of acute leukaemia, which Frances has, things tend to work fairly fast. Some cases of chronic leukaemia go on for years, having blood transfusions and so on to keep them going. These cases are usually adults. But if we can keep Frankie going on for a year or more – well, who knows what may come up?'

He was echoing the words of the Specialist. Talking this over with Arthur later, we remarked how wonderful it was that we did not have to wait for medical research to come up with a cure for leukaemia – our God could step in and heal her *now*.

Up till that time, in common with many other people, we had come to regard all talk of spiritual healing as slightly suspect. Only a few rather odd people talked seriously of miraculous healing, we thought – and the mere mention of the noisy, emotional type of healing campaign was particularly distasteful.

Now we discovered that there was a revival of interest in healing in many branches of the Christian Church, and notably in the Church of England. Some Anglicans whom we had come to know and respect asked us if we were interested in taking Frankie to Crowhurst, the Sussex Home of Healing, for the laying-on-of-hands and prayer for healing. These friends kindly offered to take us down to a private service in the Chapel at Crowhurst.

On the day we brought Frankie home, she was bubbling over with happiness. As Arthur carried her indoors, I had to fight back the tears of mingled joy and grief. It seemed almost like play-acting – smiling and laughing over the homecoming of a little girl whose frail body hid the insidious destruction of a fatal disease.

'Put it from your mind,' I told myself. 'Hold on to your faith in her complete recovery. Do you believe the Lord will do this thing for you? Then away with self-pity and morbid thoughts. Rejoice!'

And that is exactly what we did.

'You know,' I said to Arthur later, 'I just don't feel any need to struggle for faith – do you? It's there, like a wonderful, unexpected gift.'

During the days that followed, we felt almost frauds when people offered us their sympathy. In our hearts we thought: 'They're trying to show us how much they feel for us, knowing that Frankie must die. But she's not going to die – God is going to give our village a miracle! What a wonderful witness to His power that will be!'

At first, we used to take Frankie out in a wheelchair, sometimes walking two miles into Haywards Heath to shop. As we walked, we noticed that everybody looked at the figure in the chair, then smiled. Touched, we said to Frankie:

'Have you noticed how everybody smiles at you, sweetie? I suppose because you're in a wheelchair. Isn't that kind?'

She nodded – we could not see her face from behind, of course. Then:

'I always smile at them first, you know,' she said.

We were afraid that she would hate the idea of a wheelchair, but in fact, she rather enjoyed it. She would propel herself round the garden in it, and eventually we had to really persuade her to get out and exercise her stiff legs from time to time.

We also thought she would be desperately unhappy about the weight she was gaining so rapidly. But even when the mother of one of her friends passed her in the street without recognizing her, she was not upset – only indignant!

'What do you think, Mummy?' she said. 'I was walking up the street with Elizabeth (this was after she had stopped using the wheelchair) and I met Brenda and her mother. Brenda said, "Hello, Frankie", but her mother pulled her away and said, "Don't be silly, Brenda – that's not Frankie!" '

Brenda had seen Frankie several times since she came out of hospital, and had grown used to the change. But Brenda's mother had not seen her since before she went in, so she must have had a shock.

If one can imagine almost a stone and a half of surplus flesh distributed over a little body barely four feet high, one can get some idea of the distorting effect it had. Frankie's face and stomach were blown up to almost twice their normal size. Later, her stomach became even bigger, and purple stretch marks like those on a pregnant woman appeared all down her hips and thighs. At first, the lower parts of her legs and arms did not become fat, but remained thin, giving an even more grotesque effect, but later, even her hands and fingers, calves and ankles became thick and ungainly. Also, due, I suppose, to the hormone content of the drug, fine hairs began to appear on her upper lip, chin and back.

Any mother will readily imagine what I went through in

those days. I would sit and watch Frankie hungrily shovelling food into her mouth, her swollen face bulging forward from a thick, almost non-existent neck, and my heart would cry out:

'This isn't my little Frankie! Not the dainty, fairy-like little girl with the slender figure and beautiful hands, who always ate so frugally; not my little blonde, angel-faced daughter!' When I bathed her, I choked back the horror I felt at the sight of her grotesquely swollen body and purple-scarred hips. At night, when I crept into her room to tuck her in, I felt that this must be a nightmare, and that the huge, red face on the pillow would suddenly shrink, and my sweet, pink and white wild-rose smile up at me again.

One night I dreamed that this happened. That I went into the children's room and found the dainty, slender little girl who was Frankie, sitting up in bed. When I awoke, I took comfort from the thought that this was a promise of what would one day be. And so it was – but not quite as I imagined.

Arthur found it hard to understand the distress that this physical change caused me.

'It's just the same Frankie inside!' he soothed one evening, when I was sobbing inconsolably.

But again, I feel that any mother will understand how I suffered over that little body to which I had given birth, and which I had bathed and washed and done so much for over the years. We cannot help loving the bodies of those who belong to us.

The wonder was that Frankie did not mind at all. People would say, 'Doesn't she mind? Surely she gets upset when she looks in the mirror? After all, she'll soon be ten, and at that age one is very self-conscious about one's appearance!'

This, to us, was all part of the miracle in which we were involved. It was as though God was going on ahead, smoothing out the rough places, brushing away all obstacles to our happiness, as indeed He was.

Frankie would look in the mirror and say: 'I rather *like* my fat old face and legs! I don't like skinny people! I've been skinny too long.' Actually, she had never been 'skinny' – just very slight and small-boned, but I was not foolish enough to point this out. She enjoyed being fitted up with new cotton dresses, which I made in the fashionable waistless style. They looked like little maternity dresses, and served the same purpose.

After a while, when I saw how happy Frankie was, I stopped grieving over her ever-increasing weight, and even got used to her new appearance. Her cheeks were so rosy and brown from continually playing in the sun, and her eyes so blue and shining with vigour and life, that I knew it was foolish to fret.

In any case, the outbursts of distress I had in those early days were momentary affairs. The distress could never probe too deeply, for if it did, it was immediately neutralized by the miraculous peace of God which reigned in my innermost being. Going to bed one night after one of these 'attacks' of distress, we read these words:

'But the God of all grace, who hath called us unto His eternal glory, by Jesus Christ, after that ye have suffered a while, make you perfect, stablish, strengthen, settle you.'

Called to eternal glory! Beside that, all earthly suffering of mind or body must pale.

Chapter 7

I can only remember the weeks that followed as a time of golden sunshine – both in regard to the weather, and to our family happiness. It was as though God were pouring His blessing down upon us in a very special way.

When she first came out of hospital, Frankie asked for a pictorial dictionary. She spent hours sitting in her wheelchair in the garden, turning up words, reading their meaning, and writing lists of all the different kinds of fish, or dogs, or monkeys. 'Isn't life *interesting,* Mummy!' she had said, on the very day after we had received the 'sentence of death' . . . this was her attitude to everything she saw or read.

Sometimes we took her to the sea.

'Let's go on the pier!' she'd cry. 'Let's all go and have a good giggle!'

She loved the crazy mirrors on the pier at Brighton; in fact she liked anything that was good for a hearty laugh. Life was good, life was exciting and meant to be enjoyed, her sparkling blue eyes implied!

It was at about this time that we took her to the Healing Home at Crowhurst. Again, her eager little face shone as we explained to her the purpose of the visit. We told her that although the doctors were doing all they could to put her blood right, yet really, Jesus was the greatest Physician of all, and we were going to visit a special chapel where one of God's particularly gifted servants would lay his hands on her head and say a special prayer for her healing.

The little chapel was full of a quiet peace and calm. Members of staff who knew about our circumstances had come in quietly to join in the private service, and were already kneeling in prayer when we arrived. We took our places on the pew at the front, having first been introduced to a gracious and friendly Mr. Bennett, who asked simply that we should forget him completely, and think only of Christ Himself.

What followed next was a wonderful experience for us all, for not only did Mr. Bennett lay his hands upon Frankie, but he did the same for the whole family. Beginning with Arthur, he prayed for each of us individually, asking for special healing grace for each one of us, and calling down the power of the risen Christ as he laid his sensitive, dedicated hands upon our heads.

As non-conformists, the sacramental quality in this little ceremony was somewhat unfamiliar. But the beauty and simplicity of the experience, and the calm serenity which seemed to surround the whole Home will remain in our memories for a very long time. As we drove away down the little twisting country lane, our hearts were full of a sense of exaltation.

'I ought to be able to leap and run, like the lame man at the Beautiful Gate,' remarked Frankie. 'Perhaps I will when I get home.'

She was leaping and running before very long, and by September she was ready to go back to school. But first we had a wonderful holiday in a caravan near Bournemouth. This came about in a quite remarkable way, for our financial position would not have allowed us to have a holiday of this kind had not the owner of the caravan offered it to us free of charge. The dates she mentioned exactly coincided with the ones when Arthur would be free from Church responsibilities, and not only did the holiday itself cost us nothing, but another anonymous friend offered to pay for us to be transported to and from the caravan by car.

What a wonderful holiday that was! The fun of staying in a caravan for the first time, the daily walks to the lovely secluded beaches, a day trip to the Isle of Wight and a tour of Southampton docks – not to mention the cloudless skies and warm sunshine which greeted us every day of that September holiday – how could we doubt the goodness of our Heavenly Father?

Were we spoiled during those days – days which could have been so difficult in so many ways? We tried hard not to be. But we shall always be grateful to the many friends who, during a time when financial hardship could have been a kind of last straw to break the camel's back, opened their hearts, under the prompting hand of God, with such loving and giving. One of our own church members, quite unknown to anyone else – and very often quite unknown to me! – never failed, during the whole year of Frankie's illness, to slip two half-crowns into my coat pocket every Sunday morning after church.

Another way in which God provided for all our extra needs during this period was through my writing. I mention this because the measure of success I experienced throughout that particular year was unlike anything I have ever known before or since. This was another clear evidence of God's perfect timing in our lives, not only because it provided for our material needs, but also because it provided – for me – the necessity to absorb my mind at times in matters quite outside the realm of Frankie's illness. In His infinite wisdom, He knew just how necessary this was.

Never before, in fact, had Arthur and I known a year so full of activity and responsibility as that year. Added to all our other duties and church work, we were both elected Presidents of certain groups that year. Was this mere coincidence? Looking back, we are sure, now, that it wasn't.

When Frankie went back to school, she had stopped gaining weight, but was, of course, still very much larger than when she was last in school. She came home highly indignant (but quite unruffled) one day, to inform us that someone in her own class had asked her if she were a new girl.

'How stupid can you get!' was her somewhat caustic remark. It is still a marvel to us, as we look back, that she minded so little – in fact seemed blissfully unaware – of how much she had changed. When she went off one morning wearing a new pair of blue tights under the tartan 'shift' I had made to help camouflage her shape, she surveyed her plump legs with smug satisfaction. 'I shall be sorry if my legs ever go thin again,' she said.

One day she came home looking a little subdued.

'There's been a fine to-do at school today!' she said. Everybody's been crying – me as well.'

'Whatever for?' we asked, alarmed.

'Jean Peterson started it. She said, "I know an awful secret, but I mustn't tell you what it is." Well, of course that made me want to know badly, what the secret was, so I kept on at her till she told me. You'll never guess what she said.'

'Go on,' we said in a strangled voice.

'She said I was going to die!'

Our hearts seemed to stand still. 'Whatever did she say a thing like that for?' I managed to gasp.

'Don't ask me! Anyway, I started to cry, then Brenda cried, then Jean started, and in the end nearly everybody was crying at once. . . .'

'Where was Mr. Swain?' (Mr. Swain was the new teacher we had heard so much about recently. Judging by what all the girls in his class said about him, we thought he had been named pretty aptly!)

'Oh, he came in after a bit, and when he heard all about it, he was really cross. He went and got the head-teacher, and he was furious, too. He wanted to know who had started the whole thing, and then everybody started talking at once, and crying, and there was an awful noise!'

'How awful!' We couldn't think what else to say.

'I should say it was. Golly! In the end, do you know what Norma said?'

We shook our heads.

'She said, "As if a little girl with a face as brown and round as Frankie's could possibly *die*!"'

When she had gone out to play – skipping and singing – not a care in the world, we sat down and wondered just how it could have all begun, and how it would end. We were not to wonder for long. Soon there was a knock at the door, and when we opened it, there stood an older girl, who didn't even go to the primary school any more. She was pressing a grubby handkerchief to her mouth, and sobbing miserably.

'You'd better come in, Ruby,' I said.

She sat down on the edge of the sofa, and out it all came.

'Oh, Mrs. Mitson, I'm so sorry, but honestly, it wasn't my fault, and now I shall get into awful trouble, and everyone is calling me a liar, and I never said anything – honestly I didn't —'

Bit by bit the story came out. Ruby had overheard her parents talking about Frankie when she first came out of hospital, and she had heard them say: 'Of course, there's no cure for that. The child can't live for more than a few months.'

Childlike, the girl had imparted this piece of information to her friend, making her promise not to tell. But unfortunately the friend had done the same thing in her turn, and so on, until the rumour had spread, and the damage was done.

What could we say to the sobbing girl at our side? At all costs, the rumour must be scotched amongst the children – yet we could not lie. My heart felt like lead, my brain weary with the effort of concealment.

'Ruby,' I said, 'you mustn't worry about this any more. But I want you to promise that if you hear any children saying this about Frankie, you must stop them. Can you imagine what it must be like for a little girl like Frankie to be told an awful thing like that?'

Ruby nodded miserably. 'But my parents said —'

'Your parents think there is nothing that can be done for Frankie, but she is going to get well again. It's possible for even grown-ups to be mistaken sometimes, isn't it?'

The rumour soon died out after this. But we sometimes

wondered whether the incident ever really left Frankie's mind – especially at times when she was really ill. At this time, however, the thought that she might be ill again was far from our thoughts. She was going to be completely healed. What a shock the doctors were in for!

We went regularly to out-patients to see the Specialist, and he continued to be very pleased with her progress. When he said: 'Frances's blood count is back to normal now. We can taper her right off the cortisone,' we were delighted. Of course, we knew that this was regarded as the first of a series of 'remissions', but we also believed, that in Frankie's case, it would lead to a complete recovery. We were told that before cutting out the drug completely, it would be necessary to make another sternum-marrow test – this time under a general anaesthetic – as this was the only way to really keep a check on the disease.

Naturally, Frankie was upset at the thought of this. It was a blow to go into hospital – even for one night – when she was feeling so well. 'They'll keep me in again!' she sobbed, 'I know they'll keep me in!' These were the first tears she had shed since her previous stay in hospital, and it was upsetting for us all. But, typically, the storm was soon over, and the sunshine of her smile broke through. 'I don't really mind, Mummy, if you'll stay with me right up to the time I fall asleep.'

When I went to collect Frankie after the test the next day, I think that Sister once more felt that I was too serene for my own good. She looked at my cheerful face and said deliberately:

'I can't give you the complete result of the test yet, but as far as we can tell, *there's nothing startling*.'

Her tone of voice seemed to imply that certainly there was no evidence of a miracle yet, if that's what we were expecting! She added:

'It's just about what one would expect at this particular stage of remission.'

I replied, 'Thank you, Sister.' I knew what she was trying to save me from.

Then, one day, Frankie came in from school and said the words we dreaded to hear: 'Mummy, I don't feel too good.' For several days she lay listlessly in the garden, not speaking or eating, and occasionally complaining of pain in her head.

'What now?' I asked myself on the morning of my birthday, which happened also to be our thirteenth wedding anniversary. With a heavy heart I went and stood by my silent child, but when I spoke to her, she couldn't even summon strength to reply. Fighting back the tears, I went and knelt by my bed.

'Lord, lift her out of this,' I prayed. 'Please, whatever is causing this bout of sickness, remove it from her . . .' I stayed there for some moments, offering up my despair and dejection to God, and then I got up and went back to Frankie. I could hardly believe my eyes – she was walking about, smiling! This was the first time she had moved for days!

'Let's go for a walk,' she exclaimed. 'Let's go and buy some things for your birthday tea. Let's have a party!'

I wish I could record that we all enjoyed a family party that day. But after she had walked to the shops with me, and helped me to choose things for the table, she suddenly collapsed again. That brief hour of happiness remains a mystery to me. Was my prayer answered? And if so, why was the answer so short-lived?

The silly birthday fare remained on the table untouched – nobody, not even Elizabeth, whose appetite was usually insatiable, could muster any enthusiasm over it.

Standing in the bathroom, trying to wash away the traces of recent tears, I thought: 'I hope we never have another birthday-and-anniversary day like this one. . . .' But still I did not ask myself whether Frankie would ever again help me buy things for a birthday tea. The possibility of her never doing so again didn't even enter my head. For with all our hearts, in spite of the grim evidence of the past few days, we believed that complete healing was in store for Frankie.

So that when we were told that the recent marrow test showed a result that was not even as good as might have been expected, and that Frankie would have to be put on to another drug, we were shattered.

This new drug was 'methotrexate', the anti-cancer drug we had read about, and which we knew might have devastating side effects. Arthur and I looked at each other, speechless with disappointment.

Chapter 8

As the illness wore on, we had no doubt whatever that God was making Himself very real and close to Frankie herself. Her serenity and courage, especially towards the end, could not possibly be explained by anything as simple as a cheerful disposition, or a mere childlike acceptance of the inevitable. To her, the prayer-time we had each night was as essential as the meals she ate. She would talk calmly and naturally about Jesus, and about prayer; those who saw her during times of special weakness commented that she seemed to be surrounded by some unseen power, some 'other Presence'. There was a strange detachment about her, they said, a kind of untouchable calm, as though she were already moving in a different dimension from the rest of us.

This was certainly not due to any specially 'angelic' quality in Frankie herself, for part of the extreme lovableness of her personality was that she was always so 'down-to-earth', so open, so spontaneous in all that she did and said. She had a definite will of her own, and could be as difficult as any other normal child when she wanted to assert it!'

Frankie had, during her illness, two so-called 'remissions' of health, and while these lasted she was, of course, living a normal life, going to school, playing with her friends and eating at least a little at every meal. The first of these remissions lasted about eight weeks, the second for several months. It was while she was in the process of being changed on to another drug that the periods of harrowing sickness came.

When we received the news that the first 'remission' had

ended, and that the drug must be changed, Frankie was, unaccountably, feeling better. Shaken by the news, Arthur and I sat in deck chairs under the apple tree and watched her playing her recorder to the rabbits. She had always loved music, and her recorder was her constant companion – in bed and out of it. On it she taught herself to play simple tunes, writing out her own score in one of the many notebooks she had collected. Amongst her favourite pieces were some of the choruses we sang in Sunday School.

On this particular occasion, as we sat there deep in the gloom of our disappointment and bewilderment over the doctor's news, Frankie squatted in front of the rabbit hutch and played: 'I am H-A-P-P-Y . . .' on the recorder. The rabbits sat and listened, enthralled. Frankie's blue eyes glowed with amusement at their bewhiskered expressions. . . .

Our feelings can be imagined.

I looked at Arthur and said: 'What now? Do we take her to London?'

I should explain here that a friend of ours was trying to persuade us to take Frankie to London to see a certain doctor who was working on the theory that leukaemia is caused by a microbe in the blood. She was treating patients by means of an individual serum, formed through growing antibodies from the patient's blood. So far we had hesitated to do anything about this, especially as we were convinced that God was going to heal Frankie without any human aid. But now, there was the undeniable evidence from the marrow test that if God was going to heal, then He had not yet begun to do so; also, there was the prospect of this new drug being used – and from what we had seen of the side effects of the first drug, we were apprehensive of what the second one might do.

Let it not be thought that Arthur and I were in any way being naïve about this question of healing. We knew quite well that the phenomenal improvement in Frankie's health during those first eight weeks *could* be entirely due to the drastic cortisone treatment. When, each week, the Specialist cut down the dose, having made all the necessary tests, and pronounced that Frankie was 'doing very well indeed', we were not fooled into thinking that anything miraculous was *necessarily* taking place.

Christian friends who knew we were praying for divine healing had a way of saying ecstatically: 'How *wonderful*!' each time we told them what the doctor's report had been. When this happened, we would emphasize, again and again, that this improvement was only what the doctor expected; that this was what was known medically as 'the first remission'. *But* – we also believed that, unknown to the doctors, actual healing was already taking place in the cells of the blood and bone marrow, and that when the marrow test was made, the miracle would be revealed.

This is why the doctor's report now was such a blow to us. We really did believe – without any wavering of faith – that the miracle of healing we had claimed was already ours . . . At the same time, never did we lose sight of our original act of surrender and submission to God's perfect will – whatever it might mean for us.

So that now we were faced with a decision to make about a different kind of treatment, we hardly knew which way to turn. Obviously it was not yet God's time for the healing we still expected. Did He then wish us to seek help from the London doctor? Was this to be His way of restoring Frankie to perfect health? We did not doubt that God often works through the agency of human skill – but was this His will in our particular case?

At least this dilemma was a means of reassuring us about our own motives in seeking healing for Frankie. From the beginning we had said: 'Whatever is to befall us, Lord, let it be for Thy glory. This is all we ask – that we shall be a means of glorifying Thy Name in this village.'

Now, the thought that a revolutionary type of treatment – unsanctioned by the orthodox medical authorities – might be the means through which He would work, raised all sorts of subsidiary questions in our minds. If Frankie got well after having the serum treatment, all the glory (putting it very simply) would go to the London doctor, and none at all to God. No one in the village would think of this as a miracle – only as a new wonder cure for a dread disease. . . .

Only as a wonder cure for leukaemia? . . . We pulled ourselves up sharply. Surely, if we could help in any way with the discovery of a cure for this thing, we must do it. If, by allowing Frankie to undergo the serum treatment, we were being of any use at all to suffering humanity, then dare we hesitate? God's true purpose for our lives in this experience at present lay hidden from our eyes. We could only go on step by step until the whole of it was finally revealed to us, like a mountain path viewed from the summit.

Our friend took us to London by car, but this time Frankie felt ill for most of the journey. However, when we reached the doctor's surgery, she immediately revived. She stood smiling wanly on the pavement, looking eagerly around her at the great buildings and at the near-by evidence of Regent's Park. 'You *will* take me to the zoo when we've seen this doctor, won't you, Mummy?' she pleaded, sliding her hot little hand into mine. 'I just can't wait to get there!'

After the agony in the car, I would have readily agreed to anything. But this was typical of Frankie: where any other child might have shivered and cried after such an ordeal, complaining miserably that she didn't want to be messed about by another doctor, Frankie was able immediately to put the unpleasant experience of the journey behind her, and make the most of the day which lay ahead.

The first thing the doctor said to us was this:

'You understand, I trust, that I can offer you no definite hope of a cure for your little girl, but that with the treatment we offer there is just the slightest chance that she may recover.'

Arthur asked bluntly: 'Have you had cures?'

The doctor hesitated for a moment. 'It is impossible to

answer that question. You see, we have only been practising this treatment for about two years, and that unfortunately is not a long enough period of time in which to judge of its success. If you agree to try the treatment, you will be taking part in an experiment. I want you to understand that, before we go any further. The drug treatment you are having now offers no hope at all of a recovery. We offer a hope – however slender that hope may be. More than that I cannot say.'

We finally agreed that a specimen of Frankie's blood should be taken, and that we should then go home and consider the whole question in the light of what we had been told, and then let the doctor know our decision.

She was a most charming and gracious person, and we were immediately satisfied that we had not fallen into the hands of a feckless character intent only on making money out of other people's misfortunes.

And what of Frankie throughout all this? She was taking her usual lively interest in all that was going on, and though, of course, we made sure she did not hear any part of the conversation relating to the nature of her disease, or the fact of its being considered incurable, we explained as nearly as we could just why we had come up to see this doctor at all.

Though the young man who took the blood sample was considerably less expert with his needle than our own Mr. Hood, Frankie made no complaint. As soon as we were outside, she said gaily: 'Well, that's that! Now for the zoo!'

Arthur returned home in our friend's car, but first they dropped Frankie and me off at the North Entrance of the zoo, Frankie having assured us firmly that *of course* she could manage the train journey home! No one could feel preoccupied or anxious in her company for long, especially on a jaunt of this kind. She enjoyed every minute of that afternoon, lingering longingly in the reptile house – she was always fascinated by anything creepy or horrific! – and gazing adoringly at the bulging heads of the hippopotami as they wallowed in the humid mud of the elephant house.

When we arrived home, the whole story of the zoo visit had to be recounted to Daddy and Elizabeth.

'How did you get on at the doctor's?' Elizabeth asked solicitously.

'Oh, I've forgotten all about *that*!' was the reply. 'All right, I suppose. . . . But, Liz, this chimp at the tea-party – he actually pushed the keeper off the table – and then d'you know what the keeper did —?' Monkeys, always her favourite kind of animal (she had several toy ones which she adored), were the main topic of conversation for several days!

The following Sunday we were due to have our Harvest Thanksgiving Services. The children looked forward to all the special activities at the church, and Frankie, especially, loved the Harvest Services. On the Saturday, she helped to decorate the church, piling up little pyramids of potatoes and apples, and joining in the general merriment of the occasion. Then, suddenly, I missed her. Going indoors, I found Arthur, who said that Frankie had come in and said she would lie on the bed for a little while. This was most unusual, as she normally hated going to bed in the daytime. I found her lying on her bed, staring at the ceiling.

'What's the matter, darling?' I asked fearfully.

'Oh, nothing,' she sighed. And thinking that she might just want to be left alone for a bit, I went downstairs again. Later, she came down and asked Arthur if she could borrow his felt pens to draw and write with. She ate a little dinner, but was quiet and preoccupied. While I was washing up she brought a square of paper and laid it beside me on the draining board. Turning it over, I read, in her large, felt-pen scrawl: 'Dear Mummy, I love you very much. Love Frances X X X.'

Frankie herself went across to the church while I was reading it, and as she did so, Elizabeth came through the kitchen. She looked over my shoulder at the note, tossed her head, sister-like, and exclaimed simply: 'Daft!' Then she went out.

With trembling hand, I picked up the precious note and put it into my handbag. Just as I did so, Arthur came into the kitchen. He had received a similar communication, only his had been sealed inside an envelope. Our eyes met, and dumbly we asked each other the same question:

'If anything should happen to her, how shall we bear to look at these?'

As Arthur placed his love letter inside his waistcoat pocket, Frankie came slowly into the kitchen again.

'I feel rotten,' she said.

The next day, it was obvious that Frankie was much worse. Bitterly disappointed that she would not be able to go to the Harvest Services, she lay miserably in bed and gave way to an unusual bout of self-pity.

'Why is it always me?' she sobbed. 'Elizabeth is never ill. Never! I'm fed up!'

On Monday morning we carried her into out-patients wrapped in a blanket. Everybody knew us here; we were familiar figures to the nurses who were on duty for this surgery, and to the girl at the reception desk. When they saw that Frankie wasn't able to give them her usual radiant smile, they looked at us with sad, compassionate eyes. We were quite unprepared for what the Specialist had to say.

'I'm afraid,' he said, 'that we must get her into the children's hospital at Brighton. Nurse, get an ambulance straight away.'

'Can't she stay here, doctor?' I pleaded. 'Her greatest dread is that she might be separated from me. She'll feel so far from home at Brighton!'

The Specialist was a most compassionate, sympathetic man, and I always felt that he had a soft spot for Frankie. He would often put out his arms in welcome when she came in to see him, and usually had some comment to make about her smile or her sparkling eyes. Now, he shook his head gently.

'I must have her where I can keep an eye on her for a few days. She is very sick, and the new drug doesn't seem to be suiting her too well. Don't worry – if she frets, we can make arrangements for you to stay in the Royal Alexandra with her.'

Frankie was, in fact, so upset at the prospect of another stay in hospital – and a big, strange hospital at that – that I could not bear to leave her. A kindly Sister said that she would find me a bed somewhere in the hospital, though I little realized how difficult this would make things at times, and later, I doubted the wisdom of staying. At the time, however, it was the only thing to do, and with a heavy heart, I bade good-bye to Arthur.

But later, as I walked out of the hospital towards the sea to get some lunch, the heaviness of heart began to dissolve. A spicy wind came up to meet me, and a flurry of autumn leaves rose up around me as I turned the corner. Logically, I knew I should be feeling pretty well at the end of my tether. The strain of the week-end, and the emotional upheaval of the morning, had left me feeling weak and drained. Yet, in spite of this, I experienced now a sudden upsurge of serenity.

As I walked, I asked myself what the next step was. Where were our hopes of healing now? What had God in store for us in the coming days? I longed for Arthur, and wished with all my heart that he had not had to hurry home to fulfil an afternoon engagement. And yet . . . in spite of everything, there was this unaccountable sense of exaltation again. The Lord was so close in that moment, I felt I could have put out a hand and touched Him. I thought: *'Closer than breathing, nearer than hands or feet . . .'*

Chapter 9

I suppose the time that Frankie spent in the Royal Alexandra Hospital for Sick Children in Brighton was, for us all, the most distressing period of that whole year. Yet, looking back to those days now, we do not recoil with horror at the memory of them; and when, as we often do, we walk through the streets of Brighton, which were to become so familiar to us during those days, we remember, not the tragedy, but the triumph – not the mental sufferings, but the 'peace past understanding' which was ours at that time.

This 'peace' of which we had so often spoken in earlier days, became a living reality to us as we passed through the mental torture which is inevitable with a situation such as that in which we found ourselves. It was precisely because this experience cannot be put into words that St. Paul described it as 'the peace of God which passeth all undertanding'. On the face of it, such experience is quite illogical. How could human beings, undergoing the extreme strains and stresses of a family tragedy such as ours know 'peace of mind'?' This was the question which had niggled so persistently in my mind in the years preceding Frankie's illness. Secretly, I had cried: 'How can these things be?'

Now I knew. Not because I had been convinced by arguments, nor even because I had seen or read of it happening in the lives of others – but because God had stepped into the very centre of my life and made the experience my own. And when God does this for us, we can never be the same again.

One of the things which the unbeliever will classify as 'coincidence', but which we knew to have quite another explanation, was that the Sister in charge of the ward where Frankie was, turned out to be a Christian. So also were at least two of the young nurses with whom we came into regular contact. So from the very first day we felt we were not strangers there.

When Sister said that she had put me in a bed in the physiotherapy department, Frankie was not sure whether to be glad or sorry. 'Why can't you sleep in here?' she wanted to know. 'There are plenty of empty beds!'

I should add that for the past two or three weeks, Frankie had been sleeping with me. She had begun to have disturbing dreams, and the only way in which we could persuade her to go to bed at all was to allow her to sleep in our bed. So, for the period immediately preceding this stay in hospital, she had hardly left my side, day or night. This complete dependence upon me, while I would not have had it any other way, was at times a severe strain on me emotionally. Now, in this big, strange hospital, this need for physical contact with me reached its peak.

It was only with great difficulty that I managed to escape from her bedside that first night of our stay. The physiotherapy department was a large, hollow-sounding room, full of strange, sheet-covered objects, dejected-looking dolls, and sundry walking-aids. Up one end, in a kind of curtained-off cubicle, someone had made me up a very comfortable bed. I lay in my strange bedroom, with the lamplight blinking outside the windows, thinking of Arthur and Elizabeth at home, and of the lonely little figure I had left lying wide-eyed with fear in the near-by ward.

Each day I would be in the ward from seven in the morning until seven at night, with perhaps two or three short breaks for meals, or when Arthur was able to relieve me. Frankie had at this time almost completely lost her cheerful smile, and her innate determination to make the best of an unpleasant situation. This, of course, was due to her extremely weak condition – as were endless fears about daily routine, and her dread of being separated from me.

When after a few days, I was told that she would have to have another sternum-marrow test, as the doctor feared a further deterioration in her condition, we were dismayed. Arthur and I were both there when the result came through. As the Specialist beckoned us both to follow him into Sister's office, we wondered just how much more our quivering nerves and quaking stomachs would take of this sort of suspense. Yet, paradoxically, at the same time, underneath the scratching torture of human dread, lay the untouchable oasis of calm, the unshakeable awareness of a hidden strength which would never let us go.

'I am afraid,' began the gentle-voiced doctor gravely, 'that the marrow shows a further deterioration in Frances's condition. Her blood count has dropped right down again, and at the moment she is still not responding to the new drug. I'm sorry . . .'

That night I was sleeping in the nurses' sick-bay. Up on the first floor, with a little room all to myself and a view looking right over the rooftops to the sea, I lay in bed and asked myself, 'What now?' I opened my Bible and began to read from the Psalms. Immediately, the presence of God seemed to fill the room, and a great peace settled down upon me. So still our prayers were not answered? So Frankie was not better, but worse? So the Specialist had spoken with the gravest concern in his voice? What now of our faith in healing? God Himself spoke from the pages of His word:

The Lord hear thee in the day of trouble;
the name of the God of Jacob defend thee;
send thee help from the sanctuary
and strengthen thee out of Zion . . .
grant thee according to thine own heart
and fulfil all thy counsel.
We will rejoice in thy salvation
and in the name of our God we will set up our banners:
Thy Lord fulfil all thy petitions.
Now know I that the Lord saveth His anointed;

He will hear from his holy heaven,
with the saving strength of his right hand.
Some trust in chariots, and some in horses:
but we will remember the name of the Lord our God.

First thing in the morning I was down at the telephone kiosk, half-way down the hill which led to the sea (as I was every morning), and the usual exchange of questions and answers were going backwards and forwards between Arthur and me. Then:

'Darling, when you put down the receiver, read Psalm twenty.'

There was a funny sound like a gasp at the other end of the line.

'Psalm twenty? I have been!' exclaimed Arthur incredulously. 'Last night in bed, and again this morning . . .'

Why did we both choose to read Psalm twenty – both at about the very same hour? Both had simply opened our Bibles at random, seeking God's face, needing so desperately a word from Himself. . . .

Now, as I climbed the hill again, my heart was singing in spite of the burden it bore. I thought:

'If healing had come during those first weeks when we most expected it, that would have been too easy. It was easy to believe that she was being cured when her health and her happiness were so good – so fantastically good. But now, now that all evidence of improvement has gone, now that an actual deterioration has set in – now is the time to believe! "Is anything too hard for the Lord?" No, nothing! Some may trust in horses, and some in chariots, but we – we will remember the name of the Lord our God!'

My problem of how to get away for a night in order to go home and see to things there was solved for me one day when Sister told me regretfully that there were no beds at all available for me that night, as several of the nurses were sick, and even the physiotherapy department was occupied.

When I broke the news to Frankie, she was inconsolable. In vain I argued that Elizabeth and Daddy must have me for just one night; that in any case there just was not one bed for me to sleep in. . . . I shall never forget that evening, for it is branded upon my heart for ever. I sat by her bed, reading to her until about half an hour before my train was due to leave the station. Then, quietly, I put the book away in her locker, and closed my eyes to say our usual nightly prayers together. All the time she lay there, unmoving, her big blue eyes filled with terror, darting a glance now and then around the big, dimly lit ward, then back again at my face.

'Look at little Sally.' I whispered, 'such a tiny girl, but she hasn't got her Mummy with her. Nobody but you is allowed to have her Mummy with her so much of the time!' Three-year-old Sally peeped over the top of her sheet at the mention of her name, and I turned to smile at her. The next moment, Frankie had flung her arms around my neck, quivering and clinging. She did not cry, but began to talk in low, urgent, almost adult tones, begging, imploring me not to go.

'All these other children,' she said, 'can't possibly love their mothers as much as I love you. *They can't possibly*. It's because I love you so much that I must have you with me all the time. You can't know how much I love you . . .'

I enfolded her in my arms. 'I know you do, my darling, I do know. But you must see that I just can't stay tonight; and remember, we've asked Jesus to be very close to you all the time. He'll never leave you. When I have gone, just close your eyes, and the next thing you know it will be morning, and I'll be coming into the ward again —'

But as I moved to disengage myself from her arms, she clung all the harder, and now her little hands were stroking my face and neck, feeling my eyes, my mouth, my chin, my hair, as though to absorb every part of me into herself. . . . The desperate, groping, pleading little hands were more than I could bear: yet I must go – now, or I would miss my train. . . .

How I got out of that ward I shall never know. I only remember tiptoeing up the length of it, my eyes blinded with tears, my throat choking with pent-up agony, nodding in the direction of the night-nurse writing placidly under the lamp at the desk by the door, going out into the sharp night air, and turning down towards the station into the teeth of an autumn wind. Below me, the lights of a thousand houses rose in tier after tier on the distant slopes, twinkling coldly against the dark sky. . . . And I felt that my heart was breaking, breaking for the warm, clinging hands of my little one, whom I was sure, in that moment, I had wickedly betrayed and forsaken. . . .

Sister was so concerned to do something to overcome Frankie's depression, that when Frankie asked if she could have her bed moved out on to the veranda, where five or six children who needed to be kept clear of infection had their beds, she promised that she would see what she could do.

No children's ward is a particularly pleasant place in which to be all day. In the larger children's hospitals, they can be extremely depressing for those who are unaccustomed to seeing children who are seriously ill. Although Frankie had always been intensely interested in other children's illnesses and troubles – so much so, that in the little country hospital she had known the history of every other case in the ward, and watched with interest their daily progress or otherwise – yet in this huge ward, with her own condition so low, the sight of other children's faces around her sometimes had almost the opposite effect.

But in the bed opposite was a little girl who had been unconscious for several weeks. She lay there like a great golden-haired doll, her blue eyes wide open, and staring blankly upward, a tube often in her nose to give the sustenance necessary to keep her alive. When Frankie was strong enough to get out of bed, she would ask me to take her over to look at this little girl. She would gaze down at the little wax-like figure and say: 'Poor little Kim. I do hope she'll wake up soon.'

Kim's mother used to come every day and sit by the bed of her little girl, talking to her in soft tones, begging her to wake up and speak to her. She was a Catholic, and we had many chats together during those long days in the ward. Kim's mother told me that she believed that by sitting daily by the cot of her little girl (she was an only child) some of her own faith would communicate itself somehow to the unconscious little soul, and that she would one day recover. Whether little Kim ever did wake up from her long sleep, I never knew, but I did know that the hospital staff held out very little hope for her.

Once, Kim's father came in to see her. He stayed a little while, gazing down in mute agony at the sleeping infant, then turned away from the cot with stark grief distorting his big, manly face. The mother of the child went on sitting quietly by the cot for a long time after the husband had left.

It was this woman who later told me that there was a boy of twelve on the veranda who was 'in the last stages of leukaemia'. When Frankie said that she would like to go on the veranda, I at first tried to dissuade her. I dreaded having to see this boy who had reached a phase in this disease which I trusted my little one would never reach. But Frankie was so insistent, and Sister thought it would be a good idea, since in any case Frankie's low white blood count made her unusually susceptible to infection. So it was arranged that her bed should be moved through on the day she had had the marrow test, in the evening.

On the day before she was due to be moved, I found myself watching the comings and goings on the veranda with morbid fascination. Some of the children used to get up during the day, and quite often we saw the 'veranda children' walking around in their dressing-gowns. But I had never seen twelve-year-old Nicky, or heard his voice. As I sat late one evening looking in the direction of the veranda, I saw, reflected in the open glass door, a hand reach upward from a bed just round the corner, and painfully switch on the reading lamp overhead. A little later, a night-nurse remarked brightly to another:

'Nicky's feeling better. He's reading, and please can he have a cup of tea?' The sense of relief that this remark caused among the night staff seemed to be contagious. It was like a cloud being lifted from the ward.

The next night, I saw Nicky for myself. Frankie's bed was put the other side of the glass door, with only one other bed dividing her from the sick boy. Nicky's face was yellowish-white, and I recognized immediately the coarsened look and the facial hair which are so often the result of massive doses of cortisone. He smiled as we came in, then turned to talk to the other little boy in the bed beyond. As a nurse came round with medications, this other young lad said:

'Nurse, what is jaundice? Why have I got it?'

'It's to do with your liver,' she explained. 'It keeps on making a greenish fluid, when it shouldn't, and that's what makes you sick. Also, it means that you can pick up other infections – that's why we keep you in here.'

When the nurse had gone, the smaller boy said to Nicky:

'Maybe I'll catch your leukaemia, Nick! Would you like my jaundice in exchange? You can have it if you like!'

'No, thanks,' replied Nicky feelingly, his head by now deep in a Buster comic. 'I've got quite enough trouble of my own, thanks.'

'Gosh, poor old Nick, I should jolly well think you have. What is leukaemia?'

Nick turned a page absently. 'It's to do with your blood,' he said.

Frankie turned her big blue eyes towards me: 'He's got the same as me!'

'Not quite the same,' I replied, knowing something of what she might witness during the next few days.

My fears were not without foundation. Early next morning, when I went into the ward, Frankie greeted me with:

'We haven't had much sleep. Nicky's been crying and groaning – he's got awful pains.'

My blood seemed to run cold. Glancing towards Nicky's bed, I saw that he was lying on his side, his eyes shut, great beads of perspiration standing on his pallid forehead. Both his arms were bandaged, and his lower lip was bleeding where he had bitten into it in the night. One of the little Christian nurses was kneeling by him, gently wiping his brow with a clean cloth. As I watched her, her long, gentle fingers touched the boy's face with such tenderness, such love and compassion, that I was immediately struck by the thought that she had the touch of Christ. Kneeling there, she spoke more forcibly of the living Christ than if she had tried to use words of comfort to the suffering boy.

I could not help thinking that though her friend, the other Christian nurse, had plenty to say about her faith, it was this slender, gentle-voiced girl who personified more clearly the essence of the Christian message. In this broken world we need, not words, but men and women who will live out the love and compassion of the risen Christ. This I saw that Sunday morning as a child lay suffering on that quiet, sunlit veranda. And I thanked God for girls who are willing to dedicate their lives to the service of Christ in this way, to enter into the suffering of the world for His sake; to give, and not to count the cost. . . .

I remembered this as I tried to draw Frankie's attention away from the moaning Nicky. But before I could do so, she had asked simply: 'Will I get like that?'

'No, my darling,' I answered with quiet conviction, 'you will never get like that. . . .'

At that moment, a great cry came from the bed where the sick boy lay. '*Oh God!*' he sobbed. '*Oh, God!*'

I gathered my child in my arms and offered up a wordless prayer for Nicky, for Frankie, for us all. Sick at heart, I watched while Nicky was given a 'knock-out' pill, then, when the day staff came on to change the beds and do the usual chores, I made my escape for what I promised Frankie would be just a 'breath of fresh air' . . .

It was one of those still, cloudless autumn days when a thin haze seems to lie half-way between the sun and the dew-washed earth, diffusing the amber sunlight into a softly molten mellowness. As soon as I set foot in the street outside the hospital, I knew that I would not stop walking until I came to the sea.

Like many other creative people, I have always been fascinated by the sea. The reason for this is not easy to define. Maybe it has something to do with the essential elemental quality of the ocean, a primeval timelessness which calls forth a response in the sensitive depths of the subconscious, a response of which one is almost unaware until the thrill and the terror of it send the mind soaring to heights unknown.

Now, as I walked through the deserted streets of Brighton, crossing the hollow ghostliness of the empty shopping centre, the golden bars of the sun reached long fingers into the plate-glass windows, making the fashionable displays appear dusty and forgotten, and warming the grey pavements on which my footsteps echoed.

Turning into one of the many little side-streets which led to the sea, I was struck by the continental atmosphere of this Sunday morning in what has been described as 'the west end by the sea'. Small delicatessen shops and poky newsagents had their doors flung wide to the sunlight; a few early shoppers were already in evidence, opening their newspapers in the street, or emerging from doorways with French loaves, meat pies or fruit. An elderly woman opened her door and reached out a thin hand for a half-pint of milk; a cat lay sunning itself in the middle of the pavement, and small children wandered in bedroom slippers, apparently waiting for their parents to get out of bed and do something about breakfast.

Crossing the main road on to the sea front, I walked quickly over the cold, sea-washed beach until I came to the water's edge. The breakwater upon which I leaned was already warmed by the sun, though little pools of dark sea-water still stood glittering along the top of it. I turned my back on the pastel coloured Regency façades which stared sleepily out to sea in the morning haze, their pink, blue and yellow plaster already looking a little faded after the summer's onslaught, and moved in as close as was possible to the sighing, foaming sea waves.

And all the while, ringing in my mind was the cry of the suffering child in the closed-in veranda of that hospital at the top of the hill: *'Oh, God! Oh, God!'* . . . And I cried out with him silently, *Oh, God! why, why?* But only the sea answered, remorselessly unchangeable; dark, deep and unknowable; terrible, beautiful, majestic in its ageless rhythm of tides; mysterious and unfathomable, concealing in its depth secrets that human eyes have never seen. . . .

And I felt, in that moment, that God was like that; I stretched out futile, human hands to grasp Him and to meet Him face to face; to ask Him again, *Why, why, why?* Overhead, gulls screamed and wheeled, flashing silver in the sunlight, sweeping down on to the white-flecked waves, riding there for an ecstatic moment, in tune with the gleaming ocean, then soaring again into the pearly air, up, up towards the shimmering sun. . . .

Oh, my God, my soul is cast down within me . . .
Deep calleth unto deep at the noise of thy water spouts;
all thy waves and thy billows have gone over me.
Yet the Lord will command his lovingkindness in the daytime
and in the night his song shall be with me.
And my prayer unto the God of my life.
I will say unto God my rock:
Why hast thou forgotten me?
Why go I mourning because of the oppression of the enemy?
As with a sword in my bones my enemies reproach me;

While they say daily unto me, Where is thy God?
Why art thou cast down, O my soul?
And why art thou disquieted within me?
Hope thou in God: for I shall yet praise Him,
Who is the health of my countenance, and my God . .

Why go I mourning because of the oppression of the enemy? The cry of the suffering boy came back to me again, and I knew that I had that morning witnessed the enemy himself at work. St. Paul says: 'For we wrestle not against flesh and blood, but against principalities and powers . . .' If ever I felt the full force of these words it was now.

Covering my face with my hands, and pressing so close to the foaming sea that the water came into my shoes, I poured out a volume of prayer on behalf of the suffering world, on behalf of Nicky, pleading that the hand which had commanded the waves to be still should descend upon the helpless boy who lay dying in that narrow bed only a few yards from where my own sick child lay.

Chapter 10

When the doctor said that Frankie would need to go back on to a large dose of cortisone, I was bitterly disappointed. The one secret joy I had during those days – (apart from that innermost, untouchable, God-given joy which is the mystic counterpart of Christian sorrow) – was to see the little body I loved so much, gradually returning to its normal shape and size. It was partly my horror of a renewal of the cortisone treatment which precipitated our decision to proceed with the London treatment.

When we saw the Specialist about this at the Royal Alexandra hospital, he was extremely understanding. He showed an interest in the treatment, and himself wrote to the doctor in London for further details. Unfortunately, when he finally had all the available information, he was unimpressed.

'But surely there is nothing to lose,' we reasoned. 'If this new treatment can offer us even a ray of hope, do you blame us for wanting to give it a try?'

He merely shook his head sadly.

On the day that Frankie went home, Nicky was due to leave too. He was much better, and it was good to see him, on the evening before he went, asking for 'bangers and mash'. He talked happily of seeing his brothers and sister again, and next morning proudly pulled on a pair of brand new grey flannel trousers – his first long pair ever. He had forgotten to take the price-tag off them, and as he tottered unsteadily around his bed, collecting up his belongings and stuffing them into a bag, the large white label showed up clearly on the back waist-band of the trousers. I did not have the heart to point this out to him, and when I said 'Good-bye, Nicky, and I hope you will get well soon,' he replied with a smile: 'Good-bye, and so do I!'

Three weeks later, on the fifth of November, I had to take Frankie back to the hospital for a visit to out-patients, and I went into the ward to hand in a book that I had borrowed from Nicky's mother. I had had a note from Sister asking me to leave the book with her.

The ward looked just the same – I even recognized some of the children who had been there when we left three weeks earlier. One of the nursing auxiliaries, a great favourite with the children, was just doing her late afternoon rounds of the beds, hugging the little ones, and stopping to laugh and joke with the older ones who felt up to it. When she saw me, she came over to greet me, glancing apprehensively towards the door where Frankie stood gazing in with the old wide smile on her face.

'Don't tell me you're bringing her in again, my dear. . . Don't tell me!'

'No, no, I'm just returning a book for Nicky's mother. How is he? Is he back in? Only Sister said to bring the book here, and I wondered . . .'

She looked me in the eye, and her mouth was hard and grim. Glancing once more towards Frankie, she pulled me aside and said simply:

'He's dead. Dead and buried.'

I cannot really tell why this should have been such a shock to me. I had known how ill he was when he was in hospital with us. And yet —

Falteringly, I said:

'And little Kim?'

The woman gesticulated helplessly. There was a bitterness in her voice as she replied: 'Just a matter of time, my dear, just a matter of time. She's just the same as when you were here.'

I hurried away from the bitterness and the hopelessness of

this woman's face, and she turned again, with her falsely cheerful smile, towards the roomful of ailing children.

Frankie said: 'Is Nicky there?'

'No, darling, Nicky isn't there.'

'Oh, good. Is Kim?'

'Yes, Kim's still there.'

'Not still unconscious?'

'I'm afraid so. Now come along, pet, let's get back to the train, or Elizabeth and Daddy will be letting off the fireworks before we get home!'

All the way home, she chattered brightly. Her mouth and throat were terribly ulcerated from the effect of the new drug, methotrexate, but at least it was doing her good at the same time. She was also having some cortisone at this time, as well as the weekly injection of serum from the London doctor. I glanced at the ugly sore which had broken out on her lip, and at the fat which was once more forming on her face and body. She grinned up at me. Nothing mattered to her now that she was home.

'I don't care how ill I feel,' she had said the day I brought her home, 'as long as I'm at home with you.'

Now, as she skipped along beside me, down the hill which led to the station, I answered her bright chatter absent-mindedly, thinking of Nicky, now dead. Nicky, with the price-tag hanging on the back of his new long trousers. . . . Nicky eating 'bangers and mash', reading his Buster comic, saying: 'It'll be good to get back with my brothers and sister again . . .' Now, Nicky was dead. I could not bring myself to believe it.

Near the station, a group of boys stood counting out their fireworks. Two more were gaily pushing a guy in a home-made barrow. A few shop windows still advertised fireworks for sale. I thought, Nicky should be there in that group, his young face aglow with anticipation of the evening's din and jollity. But Nicky was dead.

Frankie said: 'Just look at those boys – golly, I can't wait to get our bonfire lit. . . . I like the sparklers best. Can I light mine directly after tea, indoors, with the light out?'

I squeezed her hand and nodded, my eyes still on the eager faces of the lads by the shop window. But, Nicky . . . Then, all at once, it was as though something or Somebody pulled me up sharply but gently. What, after all, was earthly pleasure? At its best it was a tainted, paltry thing. One anticipated it with eagerness, but somehow, when it came, it seemed to lack reality. This we do not often say aloud, for it *matters* that we enjoy ourselves, and if our enjoyment seems to fall short of our ideal, then we must not admit this, even to ourselves.

'What a good time we had!' we say to one another. 'I really enjoyed that!' But so often our words are a means of bolstering up our own uncertainty, to suppress the lurking fear that perhaps, after all, we did not enjoy ourselves half as much as we had intended.

The world is but a broken toy —
It never had a heart of joy . . .

But how many of us dare admit it?

Now, as I thought of Nicky, I stopped sorrowing for him. Why he, if he knew, would be pitying *us*, fondling our broken toys, struggling to extract from them a non-existent joy! But he – Nicky – was in the presence of the God on whom he had called on that Sunday morning when his poor body was racked with pain. Now, at last, he would understand, now he would know what we, on earth can never know – the answer to the mystery of suffering, to the mystery of his own suffering and early death. As for pleasures – was he not with Christ – 'in whose presence is fullness of joy, and at whose right hand there are pleasures for ever more'?

That night, as I watched the children's faces glowing in the light of the bonfire, as Frankie's blue eyes sparkled and glowed, I found myself thinking:

'If this should be her last bonfire night, then still I cannot grieve, knowing what I do about heaven, about the eternal joys . . .' I felt that I had been given my first real glimpse of eternity, and once more, in the secret places of my heart where sorrow might have been, there was joy – a steadily burning lamp of hope which I knew could never be put out.

It was while we were watching the torchlight procession which is a tradition in our Sussex village, that Frankie suddenly leaned heavily upon me.

'I've had enough, Mummy,' she said. 'Take me home, please.'

I took her home, and while other children continued to shout, to laugh, to let off their fireworks; while the sky glowed over the common where the great bonfire was now ablaze, I wrapped her in a blanket and made her comfortable on the sofa by the fire.

'Mummy, will you pray that my throat will be better in the morning? I can't use the stuff the doctor gave me today – it stings too much. Will you pray?'

That little phrase, Will you pray? was to become so familiar during the next few months. Frankie had a pure and simple faith in Christ which was sometimes heartbreaking in its directness. At any time of the day or night, whenever she had some special fear or need, she would slip her hand into mine and say quietly: 'Will you pray? Will you pray, Mummy?'

The ulcers did disappear from her mouth and throat, and gradually her body became adjusted to the new drug. Frankie never made a fuss about all the different kinds of treatment she was having. She went willingly each week for her injection – extended her arm, and that was that. Similarly, she still had regular blood-tests, either at home or at the path. lab., and over these, too, she made a minimum of fuss. Nearly every week we were picked up in a hospital car and transported to out-patients. The hospital car service drivers, that voluntary body of cheerful helpers, soon became our friends, as did the staff in out-patients. Frankie had a smile for them all, and they loved her for it.

In all these things we saw the hand of God – for how much

harder it would have been for us all if she had hated the treatment, or rebelled against the wearisome injections and blood-tests. It seemed to me sometimes that her fingers were constantly popping tablets or pills into her mouth – and although at one time it had been practically impossible to get her to swallow even an aspirin, she tipped back hundreds of tablets during that year without a single complaint.

During the six months following her stay in hospital, Frankie was remarkably well. She went to school, rode her bicycle, went for long walks and played out with her friends. Her tenth birthday was celebrated with all the usual trimmings. She loved all special occasions – and she spent weeks exuberantly anticipating her birthday and Christmas parties.

Her figure was no longer grotesquely large, though she was still considerably bigger than before her illness. I bought her a red dress trimmed with white, and she wore this with a new pair of red tights for her birthday. When Mr. Hood, the hospital technologist, came to collect his daughter from the party in the middle of the evening, he arrived a little early, in case Frankie was already tired out. He was amazed to see her enjoying a game of musical bumps – to use his own words – 'the queen of the party!'

There is always something extremely moving about a group of children sitting around a birthday cake on which the candles have just been lit, in a darkened room. I stood and watched the glowing faces and sparkling eyes, and as I looked at Frankie's shining face I had to fight down the lump which threatened to choke me. Going into the kitchen to tell Arthur that the candles were about to be blown out if he wanted to be there, I found him bent over the kitchen table with tears streaming down his face.

This was nearly my undoing, and typified one of the problems with which we had to cope during those days. Emotion is so contagious – especially for two such sensitive people as we are. Time and again we had to fight back tears because we knew that each of us depended upon the strength and poise of the other for our own display of calm. I had only to see the glint of a tear in Arthur's eye, and I would have to flee from the room before my control broke. Similarly, a tear from me could be his undoing. And Frankie was so alert, so quick to detect the slightest tremor in either of us, that at any time we might have betrayed our secret. It was our knowledge that this was the one thing we must never do which helped to keep us strong all through. *She* was the only one that mattered; *her* happiness, not ours, was what counted.

And those were happy months – yes, *happy*! Although much which has been written in these pages might suggest otherwise, only very rarely during Frankie's illness were we caught in a web of sadness. If I have pinpointed the brief spells when things were especially hard, it is only so that I might be able to tell forth to the world that the living Christ turns sorrow into joy, fear into trust, mental agony into deep peace. This is a supernatural experience.

By the time Christmas came, the rumour had spread around the village that the original diagnosis was all a mistake.

'It's to do with her glands,' they said, 'and not leukaemia after all.'

This rumour, we believe, sprang up as a result of what the village people saw in us as a family. They could not believe that we could be so full of calm and happiness if the original diagnosis were true. They saw Frankie walking about the village – plump, but ever cheerful – and they saw her riding her bicycle and going to school. Many have said to us since that the bearing of the whole family was a constant source of amazement – especially when it was learned that there had been no mistake; that everything was just as it had been in the beginning.

Inside our house, laughter and merriment could often be heard. I remember one evening when the girls were in bed, and Arthur and I were sitting by the fire talking over the day's happenings. Arthur was recounting an amusing incident which had happened to him, and before long, the two of us were laughing helplessly together, our peals of mirth obviously echoing upstairs – for suddenly the door of the sitting-room burst open, and the two girls hurled themselves upon us, shouting: 'Make them tell us the joke! Make them tell us! Come on – what are you laughing at? Tell us!'

Soon, all four of us were laughing together, the girls enjoying the double delight of having got away with the normally minor offence of coming downstairs in their pyjamas having once been 'tucked in', and the added pleasure of being allowed to linger for a while by the fireside at an hour when they should have both been asleep.

Then, of course, there was Christmas, with all the usual excitement of present-buying, and the traditional 'letter' to a Father Christmas in whom nobody really believed. Christmas that year was spent, as usual, with my parents at their farm in Essex, and although Frankie was, by then, back to her old habits of eating as little as possible, she was able to enter fully into all the enjoyment. Dressed in an old tweed cap and raincoat belonging to my father, she took part in a charade in which a group of us were supposed to be prisoners. My brother took a photograph of her dressed like this, clutching a mug of water and piece of bread in her hand!

After the games, most of the children in the family gave some little performance of something they could do, and Frankie played her recorder. Another photograph of this reminds me of the thinly veiled tension in the crowded room as relatives who had seen very little of us during the preceding months, listened to the sweet notes of Frankie's recorder playing well-known hymns, choruses and simple songs.

Soon after this, back at home, Frankie and I were sitting by the fire, when she asked me to find her a music edition of the hymn book we used in Sunday School. After trying unsuccessfully to play some of them on her recorder, she finally settled down on the rug with the book spread out on the settee and began to sing them. She had a lovely clear little voice, and would sing anything at any time, in perfect tune. Now, as we sat together in the lamplight, she began to sing one of her favourite hymns:

'There's a friend for little children
  Above the bright blue sky,
A friend who never changes,
  Whose love can never die . . .'

Thankful that we were alone, and that Arthur was not within earshot, I struggled to shut my mind to the words of the hymn, and the sweet, angelic voice which was singing them. But still the words came:

'There's a home for little children
  Above the bright blue sky . . .
And everyone is happy
  Nor could be happier there . . .'

I looked around our bright, firelit sitting-room. . . . A Home for little children – above the bright blue sky. . . . Frankie's voice sailed jubilantly into the next verse, and I bit hard into my lower lip. . . . I fought to shake off the quiet inner knowledge that something significant, inescapable, was taking place in this room, in my own heart. God was speaking. I think it was then that I first began to sense that the miracle we had claimed so confidently, was not to be ours. This knowledge was not a sudden thing, nor was it a negative thing. It was not that our faith suddenly failed us, or that our belief in Frankie's healing was suddenly removed; but rather that God gradually began to give us something else – something just as positive and just as real as faith in a healing miracle; but something different.

As Frankie finished singing the hymn, her face aglow with a warm light, this sense of God drawing near with a new message, a fresh vision, was only a momentary thing. It faded almost immediately.

But when she had finished singing, Frankie climbed on to my knee and put her arms around my neck. Throughout the early days of her illness, whenever she had done this, I had said in my innermost heart: 'Don't cling too closely to this exquisite joy; it may not be yours for long' . . . Now, as I pressed her fire-warm cheek close to mine, my heart repeated this warning.

In February we took her up to London to see the doctor from whom we were having the special treatment. She was very pleased with Frankie's progress, and the day in London was a very enjoyable one for us all. Frankie wanted to go to the Science Museum in Kensington, and she extracted every possible ounce of pleasure from this visit. She ran from one exhibit to another, pressing buttons where invited to do so, and joyfully trying out all the experiments she could. She was absolutely fascinated by everything she saw. We arrived home that evening tired, but very happy. Already I had forgotten my moment of foreboding in the firelight while Frankie sang the poignant hymn. Recovery, I told myself, was only just round the corner!

We always found, right from the beginning, that it was the attitude of other people towards Frankie's illness which could be more depressing than anything else. Naturally, since they did not share our faith, nor our own present experience of God's upholding strength, many took took the dimmest view possible of the whole situation. One day, someone said to me:

'Of course, when Frankie is gone, you will have to face the question of Elizabeth's loneliness. She is going to feel it terribly.'

This shattered me. That anyone could say 'When Frankie is gone . . .' was a staggering thing to me, because I honestly did not believe she was going to die. But that night in bed, I thought about those words which had been spoken with such unquestioning reasonableness, and for the first time since the very beginning, terror had me in its grip. Ruthlessly, my imagination embraced the idea of Frankie dying, of the actual preparation of her little body for burial, or the funeral itself – the mourners – my parents – Arthur, myself —

'Oh God,' I cried. 'Oh, God, have mercy on a mother's heart . . .'

Although I was not conscious of an answer being given, a deep quietness settled upon me as suddenly as the terror had come. The next moment, I was asleep.

Chapter 11

The weeks went by, and still Frankie continued to maintain a wonderfully good standard of health. She would go off to school in the mornings with a blue and white furry hood framing her glowing cheeks, and although she sometimes complained of pain around her eye, this did not often keep her away from school.

'Yoiks!' she exclaimed gleefully one February morning, 'Snow!'

And she was outside making a snowman with the other children that afternoon, enjoying every minute of this winter treat. Although her eye hurt rather more than usual that evening, we not unnaturally put it down to the glare of the sun and snow. The village children skated on the pond, making a picture postcard scene in their bright red, blue and yellow jerseys and caps, as they zigzagged against the grey ice. The coloured paintwork of the cottages surrounding the pond, and the beautiful tracery of the bare tree branches formed, in their turn, an effective backcloth, and the frosty blue of the sky was flushed with the fiery brilliance of winter sunset.

'Yoiks!' uttered Frankie rather triumphantly one day, as she bounced in from school. ('Yoiks', I might add, seemed to be the current school-girl expletive of the day.) 'Mr. Swain told me off today – for talking in class!'

I sensed this was a boast rather than a confession. To be 'told off' gave one more status than to be treated with the deferential care to which she was accustomed!

Every Saturday she visited a certain little sweetshop in the village where the lame, bachelor shopkeeper had a soft spot for her. He always called her by her nick-name, Frankie, spoken with a typical Sussex drawl, and when I went in there alone, would always inquire after her, often regaling me with accounts of what she had said to him when last in the shop. Harold, as everyone in the village called him, could be sure of a Saturday morning visit from Frankie when she was well enough to go round.

One Saturday in March, her friends persuaded her to go for a cycle-ride with them. Unknown to us, she cycled several miles, and came back triumphant, but exhausted. The next day the pain around her eye was so bad that she had to lie down all day. We tried keeping it covered up, keeping it closed, holding cold compresses on it, but to no avail.

There followed a period of anxiety in which Frankie sometimes went to school for half days, sometimes not at all. Sometimes she played and talked happily at home, sometimes she lay silently on the sofa, begging me from time to time to do something about her eye, as the pain was spreading to the side of her head.

It soon became clear that her health was deteriorating again. She was frequently sick, and her appetite was very poor indeed. We tried to tempt her with all sorts of things, and got to the point where, if she so much as mentioned a fancy for anything at all, one of us would rush out to buy it. Sometimes it might be potato crisps; at other times, a tomato – just to get her to eat anything was a triumph.

Soon it began to dawn on us that the methotrexate was failing. She was weakening so rapidly that we knew something would have to be done. When we took her to see the Specialist one Monday morning, we felt sure that he would want to keep her in hospital again. Frankie herself dreaded this. Although we did not mention the possibility to her, it was certainly in her mind, for she made me kneel down in the dining-room while we waited for the hospital car, and pray that she would be allowed to come home again.

The doctor was certainly concerned about her condition,

but said that he thought it was just possible that she had contracted flu. He advised me to take her home and keep her warm, bring her back in a week and he would see what her blood count was like in the meantime. Frankie and I walked out of that hospital on air – at least, I walked; I believe she had to be carried. I felt sure that Arthur would be astonished to see that I had brought her home again. But he had spent most of the time we were away on his knees, and quietly informed me that he knew, somewhere about the middle of the morning, that everything would be all right. It was then that Frankie turned to me and said:

'You know, Mummy, as we were going along in the car, some words kept singing themselves in my mind. Are they the words of a chorus? I don't know. Anyway, it was this: "*Because Jesus died for me, He will take care of me, all the way*".'

We looked in vain for a chorus or a hymn which said just these words. We could only conclude that it was the voice of God Himself speaking words of comfort and assurance to her fearful little heart: so that, even if the doctor had said 'hospital', still she would not have been afraid, for He had promised to be with her all the way, and told her so Himself.

We were struck afresh by the completeness and simplicity of her faith . . . 'Whosoever shall not receive the kingdom of God as a little child, shall in no wise enter therein' . . . When Frankie said: *'Because Jesus died for me'* she encompassed the very core of the gospel message. She held in her hand the precious stone which has become for so many a 'rock of offence', 'a stone of stumbling'. The cross of Christ must be central in all our thinking. Unless this is so, there is much in life that we shall fail to understand, much that will utterly defeat us. For it is only through His atoning work on the Cross that any of His blessing can be ours. *'Because Jesus died for me'* . . . this is the key without which we cannot enter in. To a little sick girl of ten He gave the key.

In spite of the growing signs that God had some other

purpose for us all, I for one continued to think in terms of physical healing, as an entry in the diary for March 21st may show. It was the Sunday following the visit to the doctor, and we were struggling to get Frankie on to the last and, we knew, final drug. But she could not keep it down, and was constantly being sick. Each time she was sick, the pain in her head would start up again, and between these attacks she lay on the sofa in a state of terrible exhaustion. Sometimes she would lift her finger and beckon me. When I crossed to her, she would make signs for me to hold my hand over her eye. She was too weak to speak, but every now and then she would open her eyes to see if I was praying. I had got to the point where my prayers mainly consisted of two words: 'Please, God! *Please!*'

That day, Arthur preached his usual two sermons, as well as addressing the Sunday School. He would come in after the services and go straight to Frankie, and I marvelled afresh that he was able to stand up and preach with such a burden on his heart. Later, he told me that though he preached his sermons without a tremor, he had stood in the pulpit with tears streaming down his face during the singing of the hymns. Looking back, and reading this entry in the diary, I know that this grace to go on was one of the many miracles we were given during those days:

Sun. March 21st. 'Very grim day. Frankie very weak, can't keep anything down. So weak in the afternoon that could not speak. A. and I kept breaking down – E. went out to tea. A. got through the services wonderfully. Under all the despair, I still feel a sense of peace. Will the miracle come this week? HE IS ABLE.'

When the doctor said that Frankie would have to have a few days in hospital in order to get her adjusted to the new drug, she accepted this cheerfully. She came home feeling much better, and there followed one of the lovely spells of warm weather which God always seemed to send us just when we needed it most. Now, although it was still March, the sun was really hot. Frankie sat out of doors all day in her wheelchair, and although she always seemed to be happier with her head down on a cushion, she was bright and cheerful and watched the blackbirds building their nests, studying up their habits in a bird-book.

One of the tests of how she really felt was whether or not she sang, or played her recorder. Whenever she felt fit enough, she was always singing. Hymns, choruses, songs she had learned at school were all included in her repertoire.

Now, for the first time since the previous July, she was not having any cortisone. I was delighted to see that most of the fine facial hairs I hated so much had disappeared. She was in such high spirits that we wondered whether the vaccine treatment was beginning to have some effect.

Overjoyed at this return to near normality, I went out and bought both girls a new Easter outfit – the first ready-made garments I had bought for some time, as I have always made the family's clothes. Elizabeth's suit was blue, and Frankie's gold, and I found two sweet little white hats trimmed with exactly matching blue and gold. Frankie was so thrilled when I got home with these purchases. She dressed up in her suit and hat, and I could have wept, she looked so beautiful. Slim, rosy-cheeked and blue-eyed, the gold suit seemed to exactly match her hair.

I thought, with a catch in my throat: 'My little golden girl . . . how long will you wear it?' But I said:

'It'll fit you for a long time, Frankie! You can pull the skirt up high this year, and next year it'll still be plenty long enough. I'm so glad you like it, angel!'

She paraded in front of the mirror, looking very pleased with herself. Then:

'Yoiks, Mummy! The names you call me! Sugar, honey, angel, sweetie-pie, darling, precious —'

I burst out laughing at the chronicle of ridiculous pet names, and the next moment we were hugging each other, kissing and giggling.

'All right, poppet – well you'd better change out of that now —'

'There you go again! And "poppet" is one I didn't count! I say, I wonder what Liz will say to her suit? I wish in a way you could have got me a blue one. Blue's my colour, so everybody says.'

'But you look gorgeous in gold, pet – and it makes a change! You have so many blue things.'

She looked in the mirror again, and I could see that she approved of what she saw. Her little pointed chin lifted with pride.

'Let's go down and see what Popsy says!'

'Popsy' was her pet-name for her Daddy. Needless to say, he was as thrilled as everybody else!

'What a smasher!' he teased.

'I'll wear it Easter Day – I'll wear it even if I'm ill in bed!' she declared. We laughed; not knowing, then, how her words would come back to us later on.

Elizabeth was delighted with her new outfit, too, when she came home from school, and that evening the two of them went off together to a school concert. Little did we know, then, that just as our fine spell of weather had ended, so this happy spell of good health was almost at an end, too. That concert was the last public appearance Frankie made.

In a few days she began to complain of pain in her throat and chest, which made it so difficult to swallow, that even a drink hurt her. We did not know then, of course, but later realized that the methotrexate drug, which, while it kills off cancer cells, also kills off other good cells, was working destructively on Frankie's alimentary tract. But I am glad now that we didn't discover this till later.

When we learned that the only hope for Frankie now was a blood transfusion, we were once more deeply disappointed. I wrote in my diary: 'Bitter blow, but amazing sense of submission and resignation; and still HE IS ABLE.'

It was arranged that Frankie should have the transfusion

immediately after Easter. On Good Friday my young brother and his fiancée were coming to stay for the week-end, and the arrangement was that we should return to Essex with them for a short holiday. We decided that, although we obviously would not be able to go away now, we should not prevent the young couple from coming to stay, in spite of Frankie's poor condition. In between her dark bouts of depression and sickness, she looked forward to the visit, as she was very fond of my brother. We felt, too, that the visit would help to cheer our necessarily burdened household.

Frankie rallied amazingly as soon as Colin and Pam arrived.

'What about a picnic on the downs this afternoon?' suggested Colin gaily.

I looked doubtfully at Frankie, who had lain prostrate on the sofa all the morning, resisting all my attempts to make her swallow a pain-killing pill which the doctor had given us for the pain in her head. To my amazement, she sat up.

'Yes!' she said. 'Can I wear my trews and jersey, Mummy?'

As a little later the car crawled up to Ditchling Beacon – (we always made sure to fit in as many outings as possible when we were visited by relatives in cars!) – the glorious vistas of the Sussex Weald falling away behind us as we ascended, Frankie sat on my knee in her black and white checked trews and royal blue jersey, her head resting on my shoulder. We stopped on the top of the hill and had our tea, and Frankie even managed to eat a sandwich and a few crisps. We were jubilant!

When we had eaten our tea, Colin, Pam and Elizabeth got out of the car to have a run on the downs. Colin offered to give Frankie a ride on his shoulders, but she said she would stay in the car But when they had gone, she said that maybe she would just try and walk to the edge of the drop, so that she could see over.

We all three got out, and slowly made our way to the spot she indicated, Frankie holding tightly on to my hand and Arthur's. For a few moments we stood there, gazing out over the landscape, and then we saw the others coming, laughing, up the winding downland path. Frankie watched them running, the wind lifting the girls' hair from their shoulders, their faces aglow with the crisp, April air. Then, quietly, she said:

'I wish *I* could run like that.'

For a moment we could not answer. Then: 'You will, my darling, you will,' I managed to say. And an inner voice added: 'If not on these hills, then on the golden hills of heaven.'

She was exhausted when we reached home. Arthur carried her in his arms out of the car and straight up the stairs. He laid her on the camp-bed in our room where she was to sleep that night, and then I fetched sheets and blankets to make the bed up. As Arthur and I knelt one on either side of the bed, and pulled the sheet just for a moment, over her face, before tucking in the blankets, we dare not look into each other's eyes.

Chapter 12

As I have said, Frankie adored Colin. Until recently, she had declared her intention of marrying him, dismissing all questions as to what was to become of Pam with the remark: 'Oh, she'll have to find somebody else!' Now, at ten, she settled for the next best thing – to be bridesmaid at their wedding! This hope, of course, was never realized.

'Come along, my old cough-drop!' commanded Colin soon after the rest of us had finished our Sunday dinner. 'We're having a colour-photo taken – and it's going to be a smiling one.'

Since the outing on Friday, she had been feeling very poorly indeed, and had hardly moved from the sofa. But that morning – true to her vow – she had struggled into her gold suit before flopping back into a lying down position. Church was out of the question – it was just a question of whether she could get through the Easter week-end without a blood transfusion.

Now, after a grim morning of sickness and pain, she allowed herself to be dressed up in her new outfit and hat and set on an armchair to have her photograph taken. The photo, which we shall always treasure – though it turned out rather off centre – shows our little golden girl, smiling cheerfully for Colin. It was taken just over three weeks before her death.

That afternoon, after the photo had been taken, we took a short walk with Frankie in the wheelchair. As we walked through the village, people turned and smiled at the now familiar little figure riding, like a princess, in her chariot with her Easter bonnet on.

We were smiling too, and our hearts were light, as they always were whenever Frankie was enjoying a cheerful spell. We had learned to rejoice, and to let our joy flow out to others, whenever we could possibly do so. Only in the dark moments, when Frankie was actually suffering, were our hearts heavy: and even then they were heavy, not with sorrow for ourselves, but with pity and love for her.

The minute she smiled, or spoke, or asked for a bit to eat, or a sip of something to drink – then the burden was at once dissolved, and we *rejoiced*. We learned the meaning of Paul's exhortation: 'Strengthened with all might, according to His glorious power, unto all patience and long-suffering *with joyfulness* . . .' Not with mere resignation – but with joyfulness.

This was one of the many precious lessons which we learned. And we believe it was this 'joyfulness' which baffled so many who were watching us in those days.

On Easter Monday, Frankie was well enough to go on a trip in the car to the Devil's Dyke to visit the small zoo there. It was a wild day, and the wind howled and whistled up there on the dyke – but Frankie was determined to go into the zoo. When once she made up her mind about a thing, she could not be sidetracked. This endearing quality of quiet determination was with her right up to the end.

The zoo was disappointing. There were no monkeys – and very little else of much interest to Frankie. But she walked around for a little while, and eventually allowed Colin to carry her – but not until she had practically collapsed on to a wooden seat half-way up the incline on the way back to the car. She was depressed that night as she said Good-bye to the young couple – although they promised to come and fetch her to the farm as soon as she was fit enough to travel.

Once more, any forebodings we might have had about the blood transfusion were unnecessary. Although Frankie was given two pints of 'packed' blood, which took about eight hours, she did not make a single complaint. When we arrived to visit her that afternoon, she was propped up in bed with the needle strapped to her arm, grinning away at the gleaming red bottle which hung suspended over her hand. I read to her all the afternoon and she was in high spirits.

The following Monday morning we were on our way to Essex. We knew that the effect of the blood transfusion would only be a very temporary thing, but I did expect that while it lasted, Frankie would be feeling much better. In fact, she showed very little improvement. She suffered the long car journey patiently, lying down with her eyes closed for most of the time, occasionally asking us to stop when the nausea became too much for her to bear – but always talking cheerfully the moment we did stop.

When, finally, we arrived at the farm, she was feeling pretty groggy, but revived immediately and sat cheerfully by the fire, determined to enjoy the few days spent in this, her most favourite of all places. We all looked uneasily at the increasing yellowness of her complexion, and on one or two mornings she had to be carried downstairs. But on the whole, she kept fit enough to enjoy that brief holiday, and we took a short walk around the farmyard one sunny afternoon.

I felt it only fair, now, to tell my mother – who had been praying fervently with us all for a miracle – that if this was not to be granted us, it was doubtful whether Frankie would be with us for more than three more months. In my heart I knew that I was being optimistic. This was a bitter blow to my mother, but she hid her grief bravely until the moment for our departure came.

'Why is Nannie crying?' asked Frankie as we drove out of the driveway, waving as we went, to the gradually receding figure of my mother as she stood there, head bowed, in the doorway of the farmhouse.

On the Monday, the Specialist told us that the blood transfusion had been a complete failure. The two pints of good rich blood had been destroyed immediately by the cruel disease. Also, the drugs were failing. Although he did not say so in so many words, we knew that there was nothing more that he could do.

'Come and see me next Monday,' he said. But we were not even able to do that.

Now, Frankie began to experience pain in her right arm. We bandaged it, and did everything we could to make her as comfortable and happy as possible. Most of the time, she lay in the now all-too-familiar state of terrible inertia. Sometimes she looked at books; more often she did nothing at all. One day she said:

'Mummy, I often fall asleep at night when I'm saying my prayers. I hope it doesn't matter.'

Elizabeth, who was in the room at the time said:

'I do sometimes, too, I'm afraid, Frankie, when I'm especially tired.'

'I'm sure Jesus understands,' I added.

'I pray at other times, though,' continued Frankie. 'Sometimes when I'm lying here on the sofa, I just talk to Him, and He seems very near . . .'

He seems very near . . . These words sum up what we all felt during the next ten days or so. No words can fully describe the wonderful sense of His presence. In spite of what lay in front of us, our house was full of a quiet radiance.

On the Friday afternoon, Arthur carried Frankie upstairs and placed her in our bed for the last time. She never came downstairs again. I will try to describe, as simply as I can, what took place during the next seven days – the last week of Frankie's life.

All that week-end she lay listlessly in bed, not asking to be taken downstairs, as she usually did after one day in bed, not asking, in fact for anything. We suggested all sorts of things to amuse or please her, but to every suggestion she simply moved her head sideways in a motion of tired rejection. There did not seem to be one part of her body which was not affected in some way by the disease. She could not bear to be touched, but asked simply to be left alone. She was able to doze fitfully throughout the day, and although she made distressing moaning sounds from time to time, she did not complain verbally of the pain in her arm and chest. She seemed, already, in a strange way, to be detached from her bodily discomforts.

On the Sunday morning she woke early. Lying beside her in the bed, I tried to get her to chat with me about this and that, and eventually suggested tuning in to the hymn-singing on the wireless. To this suggestion, she nodded her head. The selection of hymns that morning included 'When I survey the wondrous cross' and 'Jerusalem the golden', but they were sung to modern tunes by Geoffrey Beaumont.

'Oh, I prefer the old tunes, don't you?' I remarked to Frankie as I went to cook Elizabeth's breakfast and make Arthur and myself a cup of coffee. She did not seem able to answer my query, and after making sure she was all right, I went downstairs, promising I would be back in a few minutes.

While the rest of us were engaged in taking some form of refreshment, a strange sound came from upstairs. Washing my hands at the kitchen sink, I called:

'Arthur, I'm afraid she is in pain again. Would you just go up and see?'

At the bottom of the stairs, Arthur stopped and listened.

Then, quickly, he came into the kitchen. 'She's singing!' he exclaimed brokenly. 'Singing!'

At first I didn't believe him. How could she *sing*, when she could hardly *speak*? When we sing, we do so because our hearts are full, because we are happy and carefree. I suggest that it is practically an impossibility for us mortals to sing out of a heavy heart. But Arthur had said: *'She's singing!'*

Joining him at the bottom of the stairs, I heard the sweet little voice I loved so much, but which I had heard so little of during the past days, singing, to the *old familiar tunes*, 'When I survey the wondrous cross' and 'Jerusalem the golden' . . .

'Jerusalem the golden
With milk and honey blest,
Beneath thy contemplation
Sink heart and voice opprest:
I know not, oh, I know not,
What joys await us there,
What radiancy of glory,
What bliss beyond compare!'

Standing there, together at the bottom of the stairs, our taut thread of control broke.

After a while I went up to her and sat on the bed.

'Sing to me again, darling,' I said. 'Sing to me again.'

But she turned her face away. 'I can't. . . . It hurts too much. . . .'

The next day it was absolutely out of the question to move her, and as she was due to see the Specialist at the hospital, he very kindly consented to come out and see her. While we waited for him to come, I made hasty preparations for hospital, quite expecting that he would suggest another blood transfusion, or some other treatment which we could not give at home. Frankie was still saying very little, and Arthur and I did our best to keep cheerful as we moved about the silent house. Elizabeth, of course, was at school.

To our astonishment, when the doctor arrived, Frankie greeted him with a smile, answered his questions, and gave every appearance of being in moderately good health. We explained the bandages on her arm and the sore which had broken out on her lip again. He stood gazing down at her for a few moments, tenderness and compassion mingling with a conscious helplessness in every line of his face. Then, quietly, he bent and placed his sensitive hand on her head. He stood for a moment in this attitude, then stepped back brightly and said:

'There's a good girl! Now hurry up and get well so that you can come and see *me* next Monday!'

Slowly he followed me downstairs into the sitting-room where Arthur was waiting, and as he spoke to us in his gentle tones, we knew that he was not going to suggest hospital, a further transfusion, or anything else. She was happy in the home that she loved, he implied; if we were willing to nurse her, the best thing he could advise was that she be left where she was. Willing to nurse her? – words could not express just how willing we were.

As a little later, Arthur and I showed the doctor out, we felt that we ought to be shaking hands and saying good-bye to him, for we both knew that we would never see him again in this capacity. He had done all that he could possibly do for us and for Frankie.

'I'm simply amazed,' he said, 'at her cheerfulness.'

Looking back now, the four days which followed seem absolutely unreal. We knew that all we had to do now was to watch our child slowly die. How slowly, we had no idea.

Sometimes, as I sat beside her, I would think:

'It is never too late for God. I believe that even now, in our extremity, He could step in and restore her to complete health again. I believe He could re-create the dead cells, fill her with new, rich blood, transform her once more into a healthy, laughing child. . . .'

I believed this with all my heart. Yet, I also believed that somehow, in His divine purpose, God had a better plan. *Better?* Yes, better! This is how He made us both think during those last days. We trusted Him completely. We just waited quietly for Him to complete His perfect will in us and in Frankie. I cannot tell you how I, a mother, could sit calmly by my dying child, my dearly beloved, and think these thoughts. I can only suggest that the victorious Christ was thinking and living through me – through us both. For as Frankie's condition grew steadily worse, so our calm and our serenity increased.

I remember waking up each morning, after a restless night, and feeling peace literally flooding my heart. Beside me, the laboured breathing of my little one told me that she was still with us. On a mattress on the floor, Arthur was waking too. And I lifted my heart to God in praise for yet another day in which to love and serve her; in which to tend her bodily needs, and to give her the eager service of my tired hands.

Later Arthur told me that he, too, awoke each morning with the same astonishing peace. Side by side we worked, changing soiled bed linen, struggling to staunch the steady flow of poor, thin blood which, from time to time, flowed from Frankie's nose; sometimes cutting off soiled nightwear from her little body rather than give her the least discomfort by touching or moving her.

On the Wednesday evening, Elizabeth went to stay with some friends. Before she went, we told her gently that her sister would be gone to heaven when she came home again. We were amazed at her composure, for after shedding a few tears she went calmly out to the waiting car without a word. We knew that God had prepared her for this moment; that she, in her own way, was as ready as we were for what lay ahead.

That night, Frankie was very disturbed. Her little body, worn out with disease, and drained of its vital, life-giving blood, could not find rest or sleep. As all the normal functions began to fail one by one, so the mechanism of sleep failed, too. She tossed and turned – even though in the daytime she was incapable of turning herself over without help – and then, suddenly, in a cheerful, sing-song voice, she called out:

'Mummy, are you there? Dadd – ee; Are you there? Elizabeth, are you there?' The volume and clarity of her voice, which during the day had failed her almost completely, startled us.

'Yes, my darling,' we replied. 'We're all here.'

I longed, often, to take her in my arms and hold her close but whenever I attempted to do this, she would say:

'Don't touch me – please!'

That night, she suddenly turned towards me as I lay beside her in the bed, and said:

'Mummy, will you cuddle me?'

Oh, how gratefully I clasped her little body in my arms, and held her there until morning, thankful to God for this last chance to hold my precious child to my breast!

During the day, her speech was slow and laboured. She spoke in gasps, often putting emphasis on certain words in her effort to make herself understood. But the things she said were not in any way connected with her illness. They were casual comments about everyday things, school, Elizabeth, her grandad's birthday, which she was anxious I shouldn't forget. Frequently, she asked for a drink, and this we gave her in a baby's bottle.

We knew that her body was suffering terribly. But this was the wonderful thing: God held her apart from her sufferings, so that the little body which lay, at times, moaning on the bed with pain, seemed to be a thing apart – a separate thing altogether from the little personality who chatted to me, quietly and calmly about a birthday card for her grandad. Throughout these last days, Arthur and I could only marvel at the miracle which was taking place before our eyes.

Only once did she give any verbal indication of how ill she was feeling. This was when she turned to me suddenly one afternoon, and asked, in the usual gasping voice:

'When am I having another transfusion, Mummy? To-morrow? ...'

'I don't know, angel' ... I replied vaguely, sick at heart of deceptions and veiled remarks. And then, she soon began to talk of other things. My only dread, at that time, was that she should suddenly realize that she was dying. But she never did.

The local doctor looked in every day, although, of course, there was nothing he could do for her. One day he arrived just after one of Frankie's bad nose-bleeds. He looked at the bucketful of blood-stained tissues, then back at the child on the bed. For a moment I was struck by the nightmare knowledge that in any other circumstances, he would be fighting for her life. It seemed impossible, sometimes, to realize that there was nothing, absolutely nothing more that could be done. He left us a bottle of morphine extract to give as soon as we felt there was unbearable pain. Then slowly, he left.

The thing that seared our hearts most was not sorrow for ourselves, but a consuming pity for the unquestioning innocence of our child. Even this flame was suffered gladly, feeling that, in a measure, it allowed us to enter into her suffering.

Sometime during Thursday, she asked for some peppermint rock. At once, Arthur went off to buy some, but came back some time later saying that neither 'Harold', nor anybody else in the village had any in stock. He brought her some butterscotch instead, but she said this was too sweet.

In the middle of Thursday night, she began to call out:

'Oh, Mummy, take me home! Take me home and put me to bed!' Her voice was again alarmingly loud and clear compared with the gasping voice she used in the daytime. Arthur and I bent over her.

'Sweetheart, you *are* home! You *are* in bed!'

She shook her head. 'No, no, no, I'm not! Take me home – take me home and put me to bed, I'm so tired!'

'If you're not in bed, where are you, angel?'

Arthur said quietly: 'She's in the clouds!'

I said: 'See, Mummy's here – and Daddy. You're quite safe, darling, quite safe . . .'

'You're not my Mummy!'

'Yes, yes, I am —'

I think it was at this point that I suddenly realized I had had all I could possibly take. I had touched the depths. All through the night she begged to be 'taken home', over and over again she said she was tired, and could go no farther. Now, I thought if Arthur gives way, I am completely finished. *I am finished.*

But to my amazement, I heard Arthur's strong voice say clearly, joyfully: 'You're going Home, my sweetheart; you'll soon be there . . .'

It was typical of Frankie, that next morning, only a few hours before her death, she should challenge us about this conversation. She lay quietly now, looking at the picture postcard of a monkey I had bought for her to send to her grandad for his birthday. As I held it up for her to see, she remarked in a near-normal voice:

'You'll have to write on it, Mummy. I can't hold a pen with this arm.' She indicated the arm which was still bandaged from top to bottom.

Suddenly, she said: 'I'm in Lindfield, aren't I?' She pronounced the word 'Lindfield' with great care and deliberation.

'Yes, darling.'

'But last night, when I asked you to take me home, you said you would! Why didn't you tell me I was already there!'

An hour later, quite suddenly, her face crumpled into a most terrible grimace of what looked like agony. But just as we expected her to scream, the grimace changed into a wide grin. She began to shout with terrifying volume, and while Arthur ran for the bottle of morphine in case she were in pain, I sat watching with terror while the little face I knew and loved so well twisted itself into a grotesque mask. I knew that her brain was failing.

Yet when Arthur came back with the medicine and asked her, tenderly, to swallow some, she said astonishingly clearly:

'Yes, I'll take it – I'll take anything . . .'

I went into the bathroom and broke down completely.

'Oh, God, this is more than I can bear!' I cried. 'I'm finished – I can't take any more . . . Why couldn't it have been me? Why her? – why not me?' . . .

But in my extremity, I had forgotten that *He* knows our limitation. He knew I could go no farther, and already the end of the road was in sight.

Any minute I expected Arthur to break down, too. He,

who usually found it so difficult to conceal his emotions – surely now his control must break!

But the wonderful thing was that when I went back into the bedroom, he was sitting on the bed calm and serene, and the next moment, my astonished ears heard him saying:

'Let's sing some choruses! What shall we sing?'

My heart cried: *'I can't!'* But I sat down beside him, and together we began to sing some of the choruses she loved. As we sang:

> 'And the highway shall be my way —
> I am going to see the King!'

Frankie tried to join in. But her little voice was no longer under the control of her brain, and the sounds which came out were loud and grotesque. I lay my head on the pillow beside hers and shook with sobs, no longer concerned with the vital necessity to conceal my grief, since I felt sure that now, at last, she was beyond reach. But Arthur slipped out of the room for a moment, and when he was gone, Frankie gasped out to me: 'You're crying now, aren't you?'

Rallying by a supreme effort, I said: 'Darling, you know how I hate to see you so ill . . .'

How many more times would I have to make these temporizing, vague remarks to hide my grief from her?

Arthur came in and said firmly: 'You go downstairs, sweetheart. I'll call you when I want you . . .'

As I went downstairs, he followed me a little way and took me in his arms.

'I love you, darling,' he whispered. 'I love you' . . .

'You're wonderful,' I replied brokenly. *'Wonderful . . .'*

What else did we say to each other that May morning, at the turn of the stairs, as the busy sounds of life went on in the street below – footsteps, bright chatter, traffic – while above us, in the curtained bedroom, our precious child raved in a dying delirium? I cannot now remember it all. I only know that we were caught up, as it were, between heaven and earth, there, at the turning of the stairs. Earthly life receded from us, and heaven was only just out of reach.

As I went on down the stairs, and Arthur returned to the bedside, I heard him say to Frankie:

'Jesus loves you, darling . . . Jesus loves you . . .'

I said to myself: 'She is dying, *dying* . . .' But the awful truth struck a terror which was only skin deep. . . .

For I am persuaded that neither death, nor life, nor angels, nor principalities, nor powers, nor things present, nor things to come, nor height, nor depth, nor any other creature, shall be able to separate us from the love of God which is in Christ Jesus our Lord.

That was it. That is what I was experiencing then and there – the absolute impossibility of being separated from the love of God. I was staggered, beyond all thought, at my own calm . . .

Then Arthur's feet sounded on the stairs.

'She's going. Do you want to be there?'

And so we stood together, hand in hand, and watched our little one draw her last breath . . . saw her gathered up into the waiting Arms, into the light and joy of His presence, never more to suffer the dark mysteries, or the limitations, or the cruelties of this sin-ridden earth.

She was Home, at last.

Chapter 13

And now, the miraculous experience through which we were passing reached its glorious peak. If, throughout the past year, we had felt ourselves to be borne up above the tragedy of our circumstances 'on eagles' wings', we now found ourselves soaring sunwards in the glory, and the terror, and the ecstasy of this eagle-flight.

Locked together in a love which had, in itself, reached near-perfection in suffering, Arthur and I were somehow caught up to the very heavens on the mighty wings of God Himself. From this dizzy, exalted height, we viewed, as it were, the rest of the world in a kind of dazzling isolation.

We could not mourn, for there was no grief in our hearts. God had taken our sorrow and turned it, according to His promise, into joy. He gave us, in those days, 'beauty for ashes, the oil of joy for mourning, and the garment of praise for the spirit of heaviness . . .' This cannot be fully described in human terminology. Our mortal lips, when caught up on the wind of a divine experience, are dumb.

When I went into the garden immediately after the death of my child, I was surprised to find that summer had come. I was dressed, still, in my winter clothes, but outside, in the streets, women were shopping in sleeveless cotton dresses. The apple tree was thick with fragrant pink blossom. The hedges had burst into vivid green leaves, unfolding to the heady sweetness of the May morning. All around me was new, pulsating life. But upstairs, my child lay dead.

Dead? This is the wonder and the glory of it: that I knew in that moment, more assuredly than I had ever known anything in all my life, that Frankie was not dead – not dead, but more gloriously alive than any of us poor creatures who 'live and move and have our being' here on earth. When, in recent months, I had tried to prepare myself for this moment, I had been unable to do so. Earthbound, and ridiculously self-centred in my mother-grief, I had thought:

'How can Heaven be perfect joy for her, when I am the one upon whom she leans, on whom she depends for security and happiness? How can any child be cloudlessly happy in a realm where there is no mother to hold her to her breast?'

Ashamed, I had reasoned with myself: 'But in heaven, Christ will be her all in all . . .'

I had repeated the words to myself, rejecting the thought, even as the words formed in my mind. I knew I should believe this. But in the darkness of the night, in the blindness of my love for the child whom God had given me, the words I repeated so feverishly to my rebellious heart remained void and meaningless.

But now, now that she was gone, a stupendous thing was happening to me. It reached its climax two or three days later, when Arthur came and asked whether I would like to go round to the chapel of rest and see the beloved body in her coffin. Instinctively, I said no. I felt I wanted to erase from my memory as quickly as possible the sight of that precious body, twisted, as it had been when last I looked upon it, by the evil hands of death and disease. I wanted only to remember the little 'wild rose', the smiling 'golden girl' who was my Frankie.

But although I said 'No' at first, I soon became uneasy in my mind about this. What if, later, I should regret having rejected this experience of a life-time, this last look? . . .

I said to Arthur: 'You go and look, and if she has a better appearance than when we last looked at her, I'll come.'

A few moments later, he was back. 'Come and see.'

Together we tiptoed into the little chapel, lit by a single candle, and then Arthur gently lifted the white cloth which covered the simple white coffin. What I saw took my breath away. There, like a beautiful china doll, perfect in every detail, lay the precious body of our Frankie. All trace of disease and suffering had gone. The eyes were closed, long blonde lashes curled on cheeks as flawless as alabaster. The golden hair was combed in a fringe on her forehead, her rose-bud mouth – the only part of her which did not quite resemble the living body we had known – parted slightly over pearly teeth.

I put out my hand to touch the cold cheek.

'Don't touch her!' whispered Arthur instinctively.

But – '*I must!*' was my reply. And I stroked the silky skin with my finger. It was as smooth, as rounded, as pure as the petal of a rose. Transfixed I stood and gazed. In my heart spiralled a single thought:

'*This is victory!* This is triumph, not tragedy!' For Christ had triumphed over death and disease. When last we saw her, her body was distorted and discoloured by Satanic disease and destruction: now it was restored to the beauty and the perfection in which God had created it. God Himself had triumphed – He had had the last word! Satan was defeated: he had done his worst, but had reckoned without the glorious victory over death that Christ had wrought on Calvary. As I stood there, truth blazed around me and within me, like a white light. No need to struggle for it – it was there: a staggering revelation, a God-given knowledge that none could take away.

'*For now is come to pass the saying, Death is swallowed up in victory . . . Oh, Death, where is thy sting? O grave, where is thy victory?*'

I hardly remember leaving the chapel. I only remember the dazzling splendour of the days that followed. Days in which Arthur and I, shut away with our Lord on the fringes of the eternal, soaring still on our eagle-flight, talked our innermost hearts out together. I could not record, even if I could recall them, all the words which passed between us during those days. Precious, intimate words, glorious, ecstatic sharing of our Saviour's presence. Night and day we talked, pouring out together many thoughts we had kept locked away – of necessity – during past months.

'And did you feel . . . ?'

'Yes, I did . . . And I knew . . . Did you ? . . .'

'Yes, and did you realize that if . . . ?'

'Yes, yes, I thought of all that too . . .'

'I never told you this before, but . . .'

'I know, I know, I know . . .'

Then later:

'Arthur, I feel I must create something out of this. . . .'

'I can understand why you should feel that. . . .'

'I must write it all down . . . it's too big a thing to keep to ourselves. . . .'

And so this book was born – to be a living memorial to her, and to the experience God gave us through her.

As we talked on, the fragments of our joint experience, the tangled maze of our pent-up emotions, our secret thoughts, our intimate, private heart-searchings, our separate, yet somehow intertwined knowledge of Christ, gradually took shape and form and became for us a perfectly fashioned creation, a possession of infinite preciousness which none could ever take away from us.

The planning of the funeral was not a mere burdensome necessity, but a precious privilege. We chose two hymns – one to show the simple faith of Frankie herself, and one to show the secret of our own strength. We saw in this an opportunity for witnessing to the Christ who was the King of our lives. There was never any doubt in my mind as to whether we should sing 'There's a friend for little children' at the funeral. Our friend, the vicar of Lindfield, who consented to take part in the service – though he declared it to be the hardest task he had ever been given – said: 'You can't sing that! None of us will be able to bear it. You can't.'

But I could see my little one singing that hymn, on a winter's evening in the firelight, her sweet voice ringing out with happiness, and I knew we must sing it for her now. The other hymn was the one we had at our own wedding:

In heavenly love abiding
No change my heart shall fear
And safe is such confiding
For nothing changeth here:
The storm may roar without me
My heart may low be laid
But God is round about me
And can I be dismayed?

When we sang the last couplet:

My Saviour has my treasure
And He will walk with me —

we held on tightly to each other, our hands and fingers closely intertwined. Her little red Bible – the one she had specially requested on her tenth birthday – lay open on the coffin beside the wreath of gold and white lilies. As later we watched the coffin lowered into the earth, we could only think of her alive and radiantly joyful, perfectly whole, in the New Jerusalem. Never had we felt so close to heaven – never so sure of its reality. No doubt could cloud our minds that day – *we knew*. We were in vital living touch with the immortal, the eternal, the real – now and for ever.

Our little church was packed for the funeral. Afterwards, someone said:

'I have never in all my life been to a funeral like that. The presence of God was so obviously filling the place – and not only His presence, but the presence of your darling little girl as well. All around me, men stood with the tears streaming down their faces. I have never seen anything like it.'

Afterwards, we were the comforters. Everybody else the mourners. They looked at us with wonder, but we could only reach out to them from the eternal heights where God was holding us fast, and trust that they caught sight of His glorious Face through us – that He was shining out from our hearts 'to give the light of the knowledge of the glory of God in the face of Jesus Christ'.

Two little incidents stand out in our minds from the happenings of those days just before the funeral. One is the memory of a knock that came on our door about an hour after Frankie had died. It was Harold, the village sweetshop keeper, with a stick of peppermint rock which he had managed to obtain – especially for Frankie. The next day he was at the door again – this time with a lovely sheaf of pink and white flowers. He stood there, inarticulate in his emotion for a moment, then, his eyes downcast, his lame feet shuffling, he said gruffly:

'A . . . nice . . . little girl . . .'

On the card attached to the flowers, he had used her pet-name:

'In loving memory of Frankie.'

The other thing which remains with us is the extreme kindness of our Lindfield vicar during those days. Calling in whenever he had an opportunity, he surrounded us with his love and compassion, entering into, as he must have done, the double pathos of Arthur having to attend his own child's funeral in his own little church – the church in which he himself had conducted many another funeral for the folk we had grown to love.

Just before the funeral, one of the vicar's little visiting cards fell on the doormat. On it was written in his own handwriting: '*Just when I need Him most . . .*'

At the service, words were read from the book of Zechariah, reminding us that the streets of the new Jerusalem were full of the sounds of boys and girls playing there. We knew that Frankie, too, was singing and running over the golden hills, tasting joys of which we on earth cannot dream, holding in her hands the knowledge and the perfection for which we strive in vain here below.

Not dead – oh, no, but borne beyond the shadows
Into the full, clear light . . .

Chapter 14

Many people have asked us from time to time how Elizabeth fared during our period of trial. If, during these pages I have made little mention of our elder child, it is because, during the whole time of Frankie's illness, and since her death, Elizabeth has led a perfectly normal, undisturbed life. I do not suggest that she has been untouched by the experience. This is not only impossible, but undesirable. On the contrary, we believe that it has been an experience which will leave a definite mark upon her character, and will bear fruit in years to come.

But it has been obvious to us that the Lord's protective hand has been as much upon Elizabeth during this time as it has upon us. It is as though God, who had something for the rest of us to learn, nevertheless spared Elizabeth entirely from any kind of suffering or heartbreak, keeping her apart from, yet at the same time, part of, the situation.

Because of the miracle of joy which pervaded our household after Frankie was taken from us, Elizabeth could not help but be drawn into it. Although she could not possibly have understood, at thirteen, what was happening in the hearts of her parents, yet with her innate sensitivity, her intelligent perception, she was able to accept, and to become part of, an experience of divine proportions. After Frankie's death, I talked to Elizabeth freely about the whole experience, saying things to her which would have been impossible before, or since. I feel sure that she understood the spiritual implications of what had been happening to us all. Certainly she will look back in later years and remember with wonder, how our sorrow was turned to joy.

One person said to us later: 'I prayed for Elizabeth all the way through – more, even, than I prayed for you.'

I prayed. Within those two words lies a whole field of truth so far barely touched upon in these pages. For from the time news of Frankie's illness spread around to all our friends, an ever-increasing volume of prayer began to ascend to heaven on our behalf. We were staggered, humbled, overwhelmed with the faithfulness of so many in this way.

'We're praying for you!' The words echoed back to us from the most unexpected places. In London churches, Kent churches, Sussex and Surrey, Essex and Cambridgeshire – even in Australia and in Canada the stream of intercession went forth. A class of children in a Roman Catholic school prayed every day, Sunday-School children in Hove asked regularly to be allowed to say a prayer for the 'little ill girl'; prayer groups in private homes, and groups met for special healing prayer – all joined together in lifting both Frankie and us to an ever-listening, ever-gracious God in prayer.

Whenever anyone said to us 'I'm praying for you', we answered: 'And we're feeling the effects of it!' For I believe that without the volume of prayer which ascended day and night to heaven on our behalf our experience might have been a very different one. But, someone may ask, what difference can prayer really make? Do you honestly believe that if no one had prayed for you at all, then your experience of God's strength and peace in your lives would have been the poorer?

Again, we come up against the complexity and seeming contradiction of truth in this. But of one thing I am sure – God has given to man this tremendous privilege, this line of direct communication with Himself, this access into the very presence of an omnipotent, omniscient Father, this 'pipeline' to the eternal – and both we, and the world around us are infinitely the poorer if we do not put it into use. Who can measure the potentialities of such a privilege? Who can say what a different place this world might be if every professing Christian used it as he should?

Just as, through prayer, our experience was shared with other believers the world over, so, through the contacts we made in all sorts of places during Frankie's illness, God was speaking, through the silent witness, to the hearts of others. A letter from the Sister whom we came to know quite well through various visits to hospital, included these words:

'It was a great privilege to help look after such a courageous child; and to know two people who took such a blow as Frances's illness with such fortitude. Both Frances and you have been an example to more people than you could guess. . . .'

Even the Specialist under whose care she was for the whole time wrote to say what an impression Frankie's courage had made on him. These letters, coming as they did from people whose lives are spent with sick children and their parents, seemed to us to underline what we already knew – that God was manifesting Himself in a special way in Frankie, and that what others might call 'fortitude' or 'courage', was in fact, something far greater. It was the power of Christ, a light which could not be hidden.

Let it never be thought that Arthur and I were ever anything more or less than normal parents at heart. No one can ever fill the gap that Frankie has left in our lives. Do we shed tears? Of course we do – but, as the hymn-writer puts it: 'Ills have no weight, and tears *no bitterness* . . . I triumph still – *if Thou abide with me.*' This we have proved. Nothing can touch or disturb the deep well of peace which is hidden in the heart where Jesus Christ abides. Nothing can contaminate its waters. The grief that we feel at times has no power to wound deeply.

We have found that the most unexpected things are capable of re-awakening this grief – the angle of a gate, the year's first fall of snow, blue haze on the woodland, a clump of purple crocuses. . . . But there are more specific things too: a twist of childish knitting on a stubby pair of needles, a forgotten garment in the bottom of a drawer, the scrap of paper we found glued to the inside of her bicycle saddle-bag, with the words, 'If found, please return to Frances Mitson, Mission House', written on it in the beloved italic scrawl . . . these, and many other things, proved to us time and time again, how near the surface were the tears which we thought we had under control.

It took a dream to bring home to me the *depth* of the well of peace which God gives. It is no surface illusion, this peace. It is no mere mental attitude, but a condition which penetrates to the very depths of one's being, right down to the secret places of the mind. The dream I had was several months after Frankie had died. In it, I was sitting in a room, an empty room, alone. All at once, the door opened slowly, and Frankie put her head and shoulders round it. She was wearing a bright red jersey and a grey pleated skirt I had made her. Her hair was a bright shining gold, and her face was wreathed in smiles.

I held out my arms to her, and as I did so, my heart began to beat loudly. I thought, 'Any moment now I shall wake up. . . . Is there time, first, to hold her in my arms? Dare I risk it, or shall I be content to sit here and feast my eyes upon her?' The next moment, she had run into my arms and entwined her own around my neck. My heart soared with ecstasy, but still there was the urgency – 'is there time, or will I wake up before my hungry senses have had their fill of her?'

Quickly, I buried my face into the silky skin of her neck . . . the smell of her, even the taste was real . . . any mother will understand what I mean when I say that I was aware of her with all my senses. . . . Then, just as my joy reached a kind of crescendo, I awoke.

But this is the wonder of it: when I awoke, there was no aching sense of loss, for the knowledge of her presence was still with me. The joyous awareness which had been so vivid in my dream, did not fade; as I had feared – even in the dream – that it would. Exultant, I thought, *I have not lost her;*

I can hold her like that any time, any time . . . The afterglow of the experience was with me all day.

On another occasion, I heard her voice so clearly in a dream that the sound of it woke me, and the echo of it seemed to go on ringing in the room for long after I was fully awake. Again, on this occasion, there was no sense of bitter loss when I became aware that it was only a dream, but the same indefinable surge of peace – the peace which God had implanted even in the very deepest part of my unconscious mind.

Someone has pointed out that if we are 'in Christ', and our departed loved ones are 'with Him', then we can never lose them. This I believe. Often, as I move about the house, I am aware of her. Sometimes, when I am climbing the stairs, I remember how her tired little figure so often dragged its way up in front of me, disdaining to be carried. Almost, I could put out my hand and touch the hollow at the back of her neck, just below the hairline. Passing her photograph, now framed on the bookshelf, my heart cries out silently: *'My darling!'* It is not a cry of grief, but a kind of greeting, a reaching out towards a living, ever-present person. Alive for evermore! This knowledge nips in the bud any temptation to grieve for her. It gives day by day victory over sorrow.

'Not dead, oh, no, but borne beyond the shadows . . .'

Chapter 15

The question may remain in the minds of some: 'Why was not Frankie healed when so many were praying and when her parents had such faith in a Christ who is the same yesterday, today and forever?'

One friend reminded us in a letter she wrote shortly after Frankie's death: 'For Frances, healing came just the other side of the border.' But there will be many who will question: 'Why not here and now?'

During recent years, the question of healing has come very much to the forefront in the thinking of many Christians. No one can deny that miracles of healing are still taking place all over the world – usually quietly and unobtrusively – but at the same time, many questions are being asked, and often left unanswered.

What is the true Biblical teaching about physical healing? Should we expect miracles today? Should healing be taught in our churches? Is it God's will that all should be healed? If not, why not? Why does God allow innocent children to suffer if it is within His power to stop it? Are so-called healings authentic – do they last? Are 'failures' always due to a lack of faith?

There is no doubt from the evidence of Scripture that Jesus Himself taught that sickness and disease are of Satanic origin. Referring to the man who had been crippled for many years, He says: '. . . whom Satan has bound these thirty-eight years'. When He healed Peter's wife's mother, Jesus '*rebuked*' the fever. And many were the 'devils' which he cast from other sick minds and bodies. Furthermore, His valedictory command to His disciples was that they should 'Preach the gospel, heal the sick . . .'

How far has this command been obeyed during the two thousand years or so since it was first given? Certainly we have evidence in history that the art of healing has, from time to time, in greater or lesser degrees, been practised by individuals in the Church, if not by the Church as a whole.

Nowadays there is hardly anyone who is not aware of the awakening of interest in the subject throughout all branches of the Christian Church. Sick of the increasing materialism, the wearisome glorification of man, the mockery and destruction of war, and the obvious deterioration of a so-called 'progressive' society, Christians everywhere are turning to the original teachings of Christ and the New Testament Church in an attempt to rediscover something of that truth lost throughout the ages in the grim morass of man's sin and pride, and his wilful rejection of God.

But as in all such movements, extremism has crept in, and many are dissatisfied with the teachings of the 'new healing' groups. Sickness is not the will of God for any of His children, these groups tell us. Therefore, we must claim healing through the work of Christ on the cross – just as we claim healing of soul and liberation from sin through His atoning death on that cross. If Christ bore our sicknesses as well as our sins, they say, should we not claim victory over illness and disease, in the same way as He invited us to claim victory over sin through His death? The logical conclusion of this argument is that if we are not healed, then it is because our faith in an omnipotent God and a victorious Christ has failed, and not because God does not 'will' our healing. From the teaching of Scripture, and from the evidence of our own experience, we believe this argument to be false; and not only false, but a potential means of increasing the burden of many suffering children of God.

What then, is the answer? We believe that sickness and disease *are* of Satanic origin. In the story of Job, it was Satan